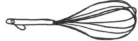

"In the tradition of *Simply in Season*, *Sustainable Kitchen* invites us to health—personal and global—in very user-friendly and knowledgeable ways. Nutrition, ecology, and nostalgia meet in simple, delicious recipes, practical tips, and useful information."

MARY BETH LIND, registered dietitian/nutritionist
and coauthor of *Simply in Season*

"*Sustainable Kitchen* provides something that googling the Internet will not: a philosophy of eating. Underlying the delicious recipes is a combination of nutritional and environmental wisdom rarely found together. This is a book to read with friends and wrap your life around."

JENNIFER HALTEMAN SCHROCK,
leader of Mennonite Creation Care Network

"So much more than a cookbook, this joy-filled invitation to engage food as a spiritual practice will inspire both the novice at plant-based cooking and the experienced gardener seeking creative recipes for sustainable living. Each page spread is brimming with practical wisdom, breathtaking photos, and the promise of healing through connection. Browse the recipe ideas, immerse yourself in Jaynie McCloskey and Heather Wolfe's gentle guidance, splatter the pages with juice as you chop and stir—and your relationship with food and the earth will never be the same"

SARAH ANN BIXLER, instructor in formation and
practical theology at Eastern Mennonite Seminary

Sustainable Kitchen

Sustainable Kitchen

RECIPES AND INSPIRATION FOR
PLANT-BASED, PLANET-CONSCIOUS MEALS

Heather Wolfe

Jaynie McCloskey

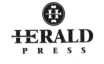

Herald Press

Harrisonburg, Virginia

Herald Press
PO Box 866, Harrisonburg, Virginia 22803
www.HeraldPress.com

Library of Congress Cataloging-in-Publication Data
Names: Wolfe, Heather (Nutritionist) author. | McCloskey, Jaynie, author.
Title: Sustainable kitchen : recipes and inspiration for plant-based, planet-conscious meals /
Heather Wolfe and Jaynie McCloskey.
Description: Harrisonburg, Virginia : Herald Press, 2020 | Includes index.
Subjects: LCSH: Vegetarian cooking. | Cooking (Natural foods) | LCGFT: Cookbooks.
Classification: LCC TX837 .W66 2020 (print) | LCC TX837 (ebook) |
DDC 641.5/636--dc23
LC record available at https://lccn.loc.gov/2019052366
LC ebook record available at https://lccn.loc.gov/2019052367

SUSTAINABLE KITCHEN: RECIPES AND INSPIRATION FOR PLANT-BASED,
PLANET-CONSCIOUS MEALS
© 2020 by Herald Press, Harrisonburg, Virginia 22803. 800-245-7894.
Library of Congress Control Number: 2019052366
International Standard Book Number: 978-1-5138-0581-8 (hardcover),
978-1-5138-0582-5 (ebook)
Printed in the United States of America
Cover, interior design, and illustrations by Jaynie McCloskey
Cover photography by Jaynie McCloskey
Photography: Rachel Joy Barehl page opposite title page and pp. 1, 7, 8, 13, 19, 23, 27, 28, 58,
95, 116, 212, 277, 294, 326 (Jaynie's headshot). Heather Wolfe page opposite Table of Contents
(top) and p. 300. All other photographs by Jaynie McCloskey. Cover recipe found on p. 69; back
cover recipe on p. 149.

25 24 23 22 21   11 10 9 8 7 6 5 4 3 2

*To the generations after me who will inherit this earth,
including daughters Norah, Helen, and Esther.*

—HEATHER

*To Jacob and Silas, who have cooked alongside me dancing
(and crying) to the rhythms of chops and sizzles.*

—JAYNIE

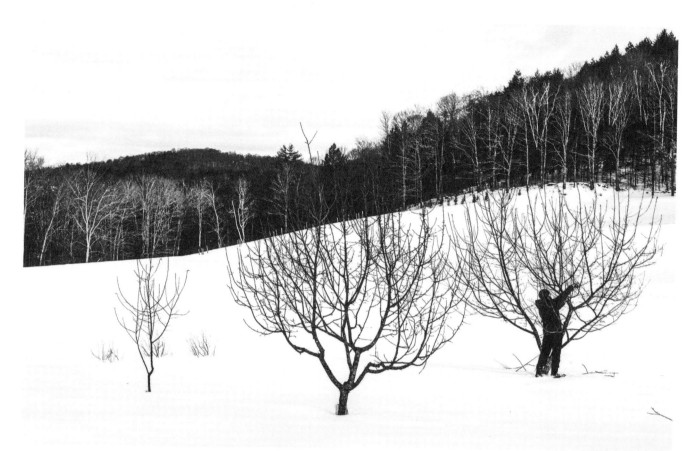

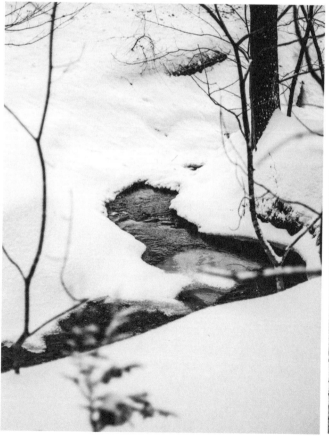

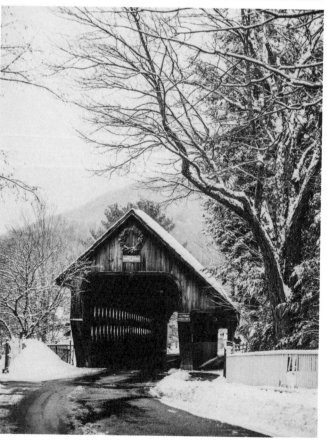

Contents

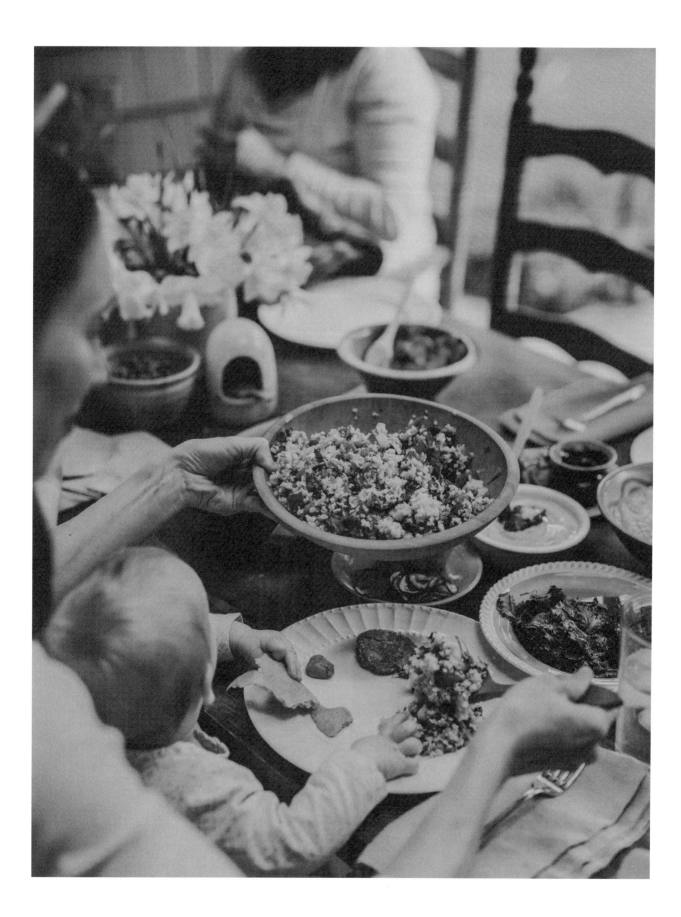

SO WHETHER YOU EAT OR DRINK OR WHATEVER YOU DO, DO IT ALL FOR THE GLORY OF GOD.

1 Corinthians 10:31

Introduction

We all must eat, and what we eat matters. Our daily food choices can either harm or help us, others, and our planet. In the world around us, so much ill health—physical, spiritual, and environmental—is related to poor diet. Diet is frequently identified as a leading risk factor in the crisis of chronic disease and is associated with susceptibility to acute physical illness. Disconnection from food—forgetting it is a gift, being oblivious to how it is sourced, eating it mindlessly—leaves us spiritually depleted. And our unfolding environmental catastrophe is largely influenced by what we eat, how it is grown, and how much of it we waste. Food is essential to healing our bodies, our spirits, and our environment.

A commitment to healthy eating, a deep concern for our planet, and a longing for spiritual connection: these three desires prompted us to write this book. As individuals who want to be healthy, as moms who want to nourish our kids, and as global citizens who recognize that climate change is inextricably linked to our diet, we are also food enthusiasts. We both love to grow, cook, and eat good-tasting food. In all these things, we experience a deep sense of peace and connection with the Source of our food, the Creator.

In writing Sustainable Kitchen, our goal has been to inspire and empower you to plan and cook meals of plant-based, planet-conscious foods daily. We wanted to create a full-kitchen resource, giving you the tools to support a healthy lifestyle for your families, communities, and our planet. While there are other plant-based cookbooks and endless recipes online, our hope is that this book makes sifting through it all and deciding what to cook less overwhelming. This cookbook is the resource that we feed our families from. It's the collection of recipes that we routinely make and serve at home. Some of these recipes have been a lifetime in the making, and all the recipes have been thoroughly tested by folks across the country. We wanted to make sure these recipes are easy to follow and taste delicious. We hope you'll agree!

The plant-based plate

This cookbook is a great resource for anyone with an interest in any form of plant-based eating—whether you are already a vegan, vegetarian, or flexitarian (semi-vegetarian) or are simply looking to shift toward a plant-based plate. Perhaps you've been advised to make dietary changes for health reasons. Perhaps you care about hunger issues and how to best feed humanity. Perhaps you're concerned about climate change and want to reduce your carbon footprint through food choices. This cookbook can be your go-to guide.

A plant-based diet is best for the health of individuals, populations, and the planet. Period. People who eat predominantly or exclusively plants have lower rates of disease. More people can be fed on a plant-based diet, as more calories remain available in the food supply if grain is eaten directly rather than fed to animals raised for food. Raising animals requires significant amounts of land, water, and fossil fuels, and is among the top contributors to greenhouse gas emissions. That means eating meat is an environmental issue. The science is so strong, the body of evidence so significant in support of plant-based eating for health of both people and planet, that we don't feel the need to make a compelling case here. That work has been done. Our job in this book is to make it enjoyable to cook and delicious to eat so that you will want to eat a plant-based diet!

THIS COOKBOOK WILL EMPOWER YOU TO

- Make more foods yourself rather than buying packaged products. We offer recipes for over a dozen staples, including homemade tortillas, tahini, and canned tomatoes.

- Cook using local, seasonally available foods. We offer a variety of recipes for each season. We exclusively use locally available sweeteners (honey and maple syrup).

- Find flexibility in recipes. We routinely include substitutions so that you can make selections according to personal preferences or what you have on hand.

- Decrease food waste. We make use of all edible parts of food including tops, stems, seeds, and skins. We offer a section on how to compost any scraps that cannot be used.

- Conserve energy by not preheating your oven when cooking. We challenge conventional wisdom instructing you to preheat, an unnecessary practice (unless you are baking with leaveners) that wastes energy.

- Limit processed, refined foods. We use no white sugar and very minimal white flour.

- Expand your palate. We have created a collection of a recipes that will expose you to flavors from across the globe, including African, Asian, Indian, Middle Eastern, Mediterranean, and Latin American cuisines, along with plenty of familiar North American favorites. We include a wide variety of plant-based proteins so you can explore less familiar options.

- Grow in knowledge and skill. We offer supplementary sections that discuss nutrition basics, meal planning tips, culinary techniques, and a beginner's guide to canning. We include recipes that invite you to ferment, preserve the harvest, and go wildcrafting—harvesting plants, like fiddleheads, from their natural or wild habitat.

- Eat a plant-based diet. All recipes are vegetarian. Many are vegan or easily adapted to be vegan-friendly.

- Spend time in the kitchen, discovering the joy of preparing nourishing foods from scratch. We encourage you to cook—a lot! Many of our recipes include cross-references to make your own staples. Our recipe for Breakfast Tacos (p. 46), for example, invites (but doesn't require) you to make homemade Whole Wheat Tortillas (p. 286), Fresh Salsa (p. 254), and Guacamole (p. 257).

- Contemplate how your food choices matter. We explore health-related, spiritual, and environmental reasons for making wise food choices.

- Connect with creation through cooking. We invite you to practice cooking as a spiritual discipline—a regular activity that nurtures positive, intentional connection with the Creator in addition to self, others, and the earth.

- Be curious about food and get to know what you are eating. Consider each recipe as an edible story.

- Share what you've learned with friends and family. A really fun way to do this is through a cookbook club. Invite a group to bring a dish from this book and discuss what you can do to make positive change in regard to food related issues.

Planning, procuring, and preparing food in this way takes time and intention. If this is new to you, we encourage you to start with small changes. Build healthy habits that you can stick with. Slowing down and prioritizing food is a lifestyle choice. We have had to be creative and make sacrifices in other areas to create a space in our everyday lives to make healthy meals happen. We have found it life-giving, and we hope that you find nourishment, joy, and reward in nurturing a closer relationship with what you eat.

Healing brokenness

Health, ecological sustainability, and connection: these are all intertwined. Where there is brokenness in any or all of these domains, the path to healing can begin with a plant-based plate.

Using the gifts of healthy, nutrient-packed food from sustainable and ethical sources, we nourish body, soul, and planet, supplying the power to bounce back. A beautiful resiliency. The kitchen is a place where we can care for ourselves, our neighbors, and our world, and by doing so, we take part in the restoration of what has been broken.

It is imperative that we change the way we eat, now. In 2019, thirty leading global scientists reached a consensus on what constitutes a healthy and sustainable diet. Their conclusion? A diverse, plant-based diet. Their report states, "Because food systems are a major driver of poor health and environmental degradation, global efforts are urgently needed to collectively transform diets and food production. . . . Achieving this goal will require rapid adoption of numerous changes and unprecedented global collaboration and commitment: nothing less than a Great Food Transformation."[1] This great transformation will be made up of many small changes. Healing begins one meal at a time.

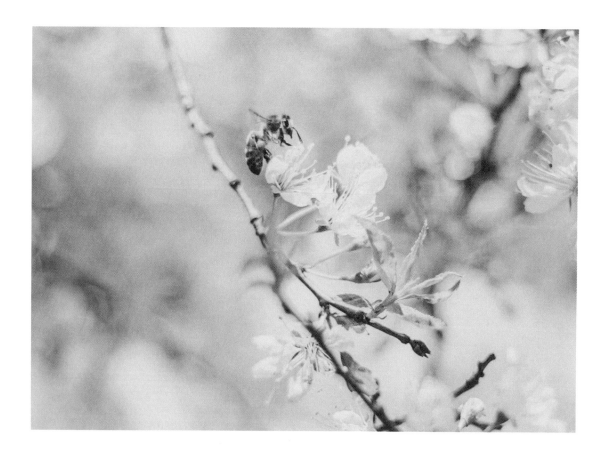

Who we are

Throughout my childhood, I saw my dad's passion for cooking and delicious food. I grew up hearing stories about his Italian grandmother going out with a bus full of other women, foraging for dandelion greens. And about how when he was eight years old, he'd ride his bike to his friend's house, knowing he wasn't home but that his friend's mother, who was Mexican, would invite him in for delicious homemade tortillas and beans. In our home, he kept the Italian family tradition of Sunday lunch, known to many Italians as the "pasta sabbath," by making pasta with his famous tomato sauce. I also remember asking my mom a lot of questions in the kitchen, from how each tool worked to "How did you make this potato soup so good?" And as we got older, my mom, my sister, and I made family gatherings around meals really fun, making every detail special, from the food ingredients to the place settings and garnishes.

While I felt that I had a positive experience around food growing up, I also had a secret life of sneaking around and eating impulsively when no one was watching. It began when, as a six-year-old, I spent about a week at my grandparents' home. While I wasn't technically alone, my grandparents were busy, and I was on my own for much of the visit. My grandparents' pantry was stocked with sugary, processed food, the fridge with imitation cheese slices, and the freezer with ice cream treats. Candy dishes were accessible all over the house. I ate it all to calm my nerves, to fill the time, and to not feel alone. When I went home, I was noticeably heavier than I had been when I went to their house. I don't really blame anyone for what happened: the health risks from these types of foods weren't understood in those days. But this started an entire childhood of emotional eating habits. I was an overweight child and teenager, and it wasn't until I was in college that things changed.

When I went to college, I lost fifty pounds as a result of bulimia nervosa, an eating disorder. If I wasn't obsessing over low-calorie intake, I was purging after eating. When I got married and received my first set of kitchen tools from the wedding registry, I really took on cooking for the first time. I began to recover from my disordered eating and I set out to maintain a healthy lifestyle by cooking healthy meals. By shopping at local farmers' markets, making the time to chop vegetables, and actually enjoying my own cooking, I slowly began to heal. I became fascinated with healthy eating and started reading all the books and watching all the documentaries on the subject that I could.

Because of that time of learning I decided to adopt a vegetarian diet, with seasons of eating vegan. I have been a vegetarian for almost ten years. Learning to cook and taking control of my health was transformative for me in a few ways. I learned that I was capable of change. The nutrients brought healing to my mind and gave me energy and stamina. And cooking gave me a daily, full-sensory experience of bright colors, engaging sounds, mouthwatering smells, and satisfying flavors bringing vibrancy and excitement to my days. I fell in love with the beauty of rainbow carrots and the taste of local, in-season heirloom tomatoes, and I was proud of my food combinations. I was awakened to a whole new passion.

Through the stress and hormones of three pregnancies, one loss, two births, and breastfeeding, I was not as kind to my body as I had been in those first four years of marriage. I reverted to using unhealthy food for comfort and relying on highly processed and packaged convenience food. This was a difficult season, during which I sometimes worked sixty hours a week while pregnant and then after the birth I experienced a postpartum mood disorder. I longed to jump back into healthy habits, but I found it a lot more challenging than I had anticipated. I needed to be able to make dinner regularly, and I needed healthy and tasty recipes that even a toddler would eat.

The idea for this book was birthed out of that season. And now, having shifted once again from emotional and convenience eating to healthy and mindful eating, I know so well that this way of life is not easy. It takes discipline, commitment, time, and energy. When those things are not present, it takes fighting for them. I hope this book makes adopting and maintaining a healthy lifestyle easier for all of us, even in the midst of so many daily challenges.

HEATHER

Food connects me to everything I love. It always has.

I grew up in close connection with my food. My mother invited me into the kitchen, sharing her culinary skills. My father invited me outside, sharing his love of the land. Together as a family we raised chickens, gardened, cooked, preserved any extra harvest, and shared meals with one another. We often ate and shared food with our neighbors, many of whom were also extended family, and with our church family. These practices have remained part of my daily rhythm, and I am now sharing the gifts of interconnectedness between food, faith, and family with my children.

My calling to a career as a dietitian came in ninth grade. My peers were reading magazines with dietary advice that was confusing and seemed to contradict what I intuitively knew to be healthy habits needed for strong, growing bodies. I was questioning and curious to learn more. In health class I wrote a research paper titled "Adolescent Nutrition." I found it empowering to explore the science behind what a teenage body needs and then be able to communicate that with others. This new academic interest in nutrition complemented my established culinary, agrarian, and environmental interests. These interrelated passions have translated into a purposeful profession, for which I am grateful.

I feel great satisfaction and deep shalom in being in touch with my food. Food connects me to creation and the Creator. I feel great distress as the crisis of climate change increasingly unfolds. By all scientific reports and my own eyewitness accounts, Earth is suffering, which causes me to grieve deeply. Here in Vermont, the Green Mountain State, I frequently lift my eyes to hills, and I am reminded from where my strength comes. As Psalm 121:2 says, it comes from the Lord, the maker of heaven and earth. My faith keeps me encouraged to care for creation in the face of environmental devastation. Writing this cookbook is one way for me to answer the question, How can we eat and cook in response to climate change?

Nurturing a close connection to my food allows me to appreciate the beauty and diversity of creation. Through our cooking and our eating, we can honor our planet with actions that restore us to right relationship with God and each other.

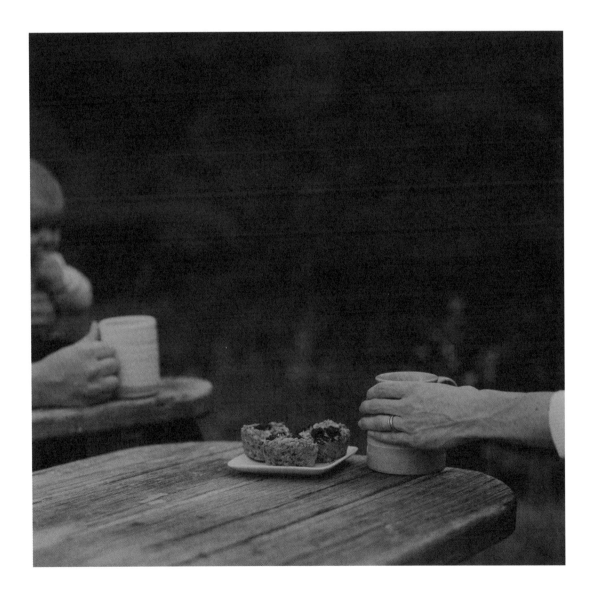

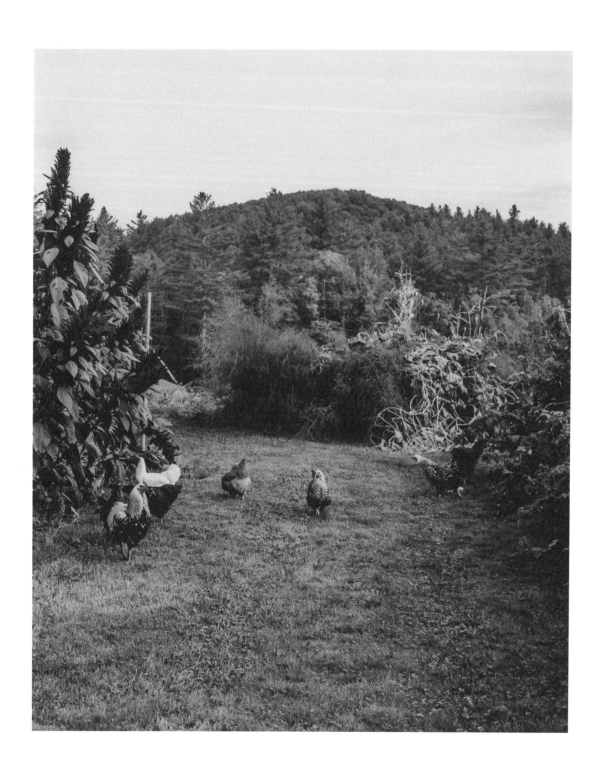

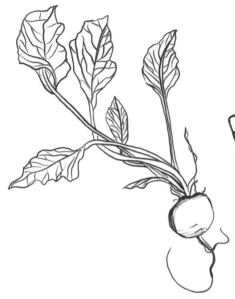

LET FOOD
BE THY MEDICINE
AND MEDICINE
BE THY FOOD.
attributed to Hippocrates

Health

Heart disease and cancer are the two top causes of death in the United States, with diabetes and strokes also making the top ten list.[2] Diet is a leading risk factor in all four of these conditions. If Americans ate healthier foods, exercised more, and quit smoking, researchers estimate there would be at least 40 percent less cancer and 80 percent less heart disease, diabetes, and stroke.[3]

Whether it is for general health protection; prevention and treatment of lifestyle-related chronic diseases such as cancer, heart disease, and diabetes; or the reduction of risk factors such as high blood pressure, high cholesterol, and obesity; the message is the same: Consume less animal products and processed foods. Eat more plants.

It's no wonder, then, that the U.S. government recommends that everyone's plate be filled, at a minimum, with 75 percent plants.[4] The Dietary Guidelines for Americans 2015–2020 encourage us to build our diets around fruits, vegetables, whole grains, nuts, seeds, and legumes.[5] The guidelines highlight Mediterranean-style and vegetarian eating patterns as balanced, healthy examples to be followed. The Mediterranean eating pattern includes plenty of olive oil, nuts, vegetables, fruits, and whole grains; moderate intake of fish and poultry; and minimal consumption of dairy products, red meat, processed meats, and sweets. The vegetarian style of eating eliminates meats, poultry, and fish entirely. Plant-based diets are associated with better health outcomes than the typical Western diet, in which animal protein and sugary, salty processed foods are routinely overconsumed.

Built on a foundation of healthy plant-based foods, our diet then has room for everything to be enjoyed in moderation. This includes a bit of butter or cream and a touch of honey or maple syrup. We use these ingredients, which contain saturated fats and added sugars, sparingly in this cookbook, to enhance the taste of nutritious whole foods. We say no to guilt and to deprivation. We say yes to moderation and mindfulness. This is balanced eating. This is having a healthy relationship with food. We invite you to develop sustainable, plant-based eating habits to last a lifetime.

Plant-based eating has many variations. Plant-based eaters include the vegan who excludes all animal products, the vegetarian who doesn't eat meat, and the flexitarian (semi-vegetarian) who eats predominantly plants with occasional meat at meals. This cookbook can be classified as vegetarian. It does not include any red meat, poultry, or fish. It does include animal products, such as dairy and honey. That said, many of our recipes are vegan or easily adaptable to be vegan-friendly.

The bottom line is that nutrient needs are easily met by a healthy vegetarian diet. Depending on where you live you may need to add a seasonal supplement of vitamin D—the sunshine vitamin. Additionally, vegans should seek out fortified foods or supplements in order to meet their vitamin B12 and calcium requirements.

A healthy diet includes a wide variety of foods to ensure we get adequate nutrients, macronutrients (fats, carbohydrates, proteins), micronutrients (vitamins and minerals), and phytonutrients (other nutrients in plants, such as antioxidants). All these contribute to health protection, promotion, and disease prevention. A varied diet also helps to mitigate potential harm. By diversifying what we eat, we reduce risk of exposure to things such as pesticide residue and heavy metal contamination. Some consumers may choose organic produce to avoid chemicals, pesticides, or genetically modified organisms (GMOs). Based on what we know now—although nutrition science is relatively young and we are learning all the time—organic foods are not nutritionally superior to conventionally grown counterparts. Of course, the decision to purchase organic foods supports the growing of food in an eco-friendly fashion (more on that later).

The mention of moderation is essential to any discussion of nutrition and health. Even a plant-based diet, if eaten in excess of the calories required by the body, can lead to health issues. Limiting our portions of everything, but especially processed foods, added sugars, and meat, is part of honoring our bodies. Moderating our intake also means that more resources are available to others. There is much wisdom in the Lord's Prayer: "Give us this day our daily bread."

Healthy eating extends to much more than just what and how much we eat. By definition, health is not just the absence of illness; it is well-being of one's body, mind, and social interactions.[6] Intention around food, and attention to our eating habits, can help us grow in mindfulness in all of life.

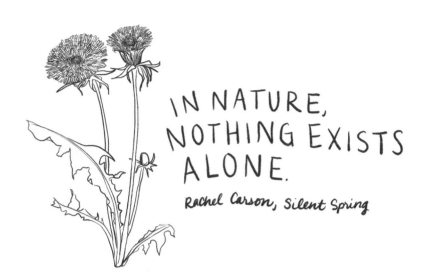

IN NATURE, NOTHING EXISTS ALONE.

Rachel Carson, Silent Spring

Connection

How we buy, cook, and serve our food has the power to connect us to others. Food choices connect us to those around the world who are hungry, to our community, to our families and friends, and to ourselves. Food choices connect us as humans to other species. And as we recognize the abundant gifts of nourishment and flavor, food connects us to the Source of all.

Food choices

When you choose what food to eat and where to buy it, you can consider a number of variables. Whatever you spend your dollars on means casting a vote for how you want the world to be. Cheaper tomatoes may mean that the people who picked them are not paid a fair wage. Buying organic cheese means fewer dairy farmers will inject their cows with hormones. Another's well-being is often at the cost of convenience. It may cost less for you, but in reality the cost is great. We can make choices to ensure we are casting our dollar votes for the best practices.

- Include farmers' markets and food co-ops in your grocery-gathering.

- Sign up for a CSA (community-supported agriculture) to support the livelihoods of the farms in your area.

- Choose a plant-based diet. This can redirect grain resources from cows to people suffering from hunger.

- Purchase foods certified as meeting ethical standards. Look for labels such as *fair trade*, *organic*, and *B Corp* (a certification that a business meets a high standard of environmental and social responsibility).

Preparation

Nature is good for the soul. Studies show that time spent in nature improves health: people who spend time in the natural world are less stressed, anxious, and depressed than those who don't. They exude a more positive mood, stronger vitality, and a greater sense of meaning. What may be a little more surprising is that the same is true when we bring nature indoors. When food preparation is plant-based, that same positive connection with nature is accessible and routine. Allowing the time and space to slow down and mindfully chop fresh vegetables is not only good for our physical health, wallets, and the planet; it is also good for our souls. When you chop a red cabbage in half, you see those dynamic and intricate bright purple and white lines swirling through it. You might pause to appreciate its beauty. Throw this same red cabbage in a sandwich with vibrant orange carrots, bright yellow bell peppers, brilliant hot-pink radishes, and a fresh chartreuse avocado, and you'll be in awe. (See Loaded Veggie Sandwich with Garlic Herb Spread on p. 120.)

Connection with nature is connection with life. When we spend time in nature, we can connect to the universe and ultimately the Creator. We engage our senses—our gateways to the outside world—with something beyond us. Cooking can be a spiritual experience, nourishing body and soul. Even more soulful benefits accrue when you add tilling soil, planting, tending a garden, and harvesting your own fruits, vegetables, and grains. (You'll also save a lot of resources that you might have otherwise used for therapy, gym memberships, and groceries!)

Getting as close as we can to the source of our food yields many benefits. Buying locally and seasonally reduces carbon emissions and packaging. Such food has a greater nutrient density and removes the distance from the source to us. Local produce connects us to the rhythms of the seasons and humbles us. We begin to see our dependency on our planet, and we are rewarded with the best-tasting food.

Gathering

Serving those we love a meal we've prepared with our own hands is sacred. Looking into their faces as we eat together and listen to their stories is sacred. Gathering around food is a way to love our neighbor. And our neighbors go beyond those we may already call friends or family. Food can connect us to those we do not yet know. Gathering around a table, we can put differences aside and unite around this thing we all have in common: the need for and enjoyment of food. Food connects us across cultures, genders, economic classes, ages, religions, abilities, and legal status. We all eat.

When our families gather around our tables, we take a moment before eating to be thankful to God and to sing together. We share our songs with you on the next page.

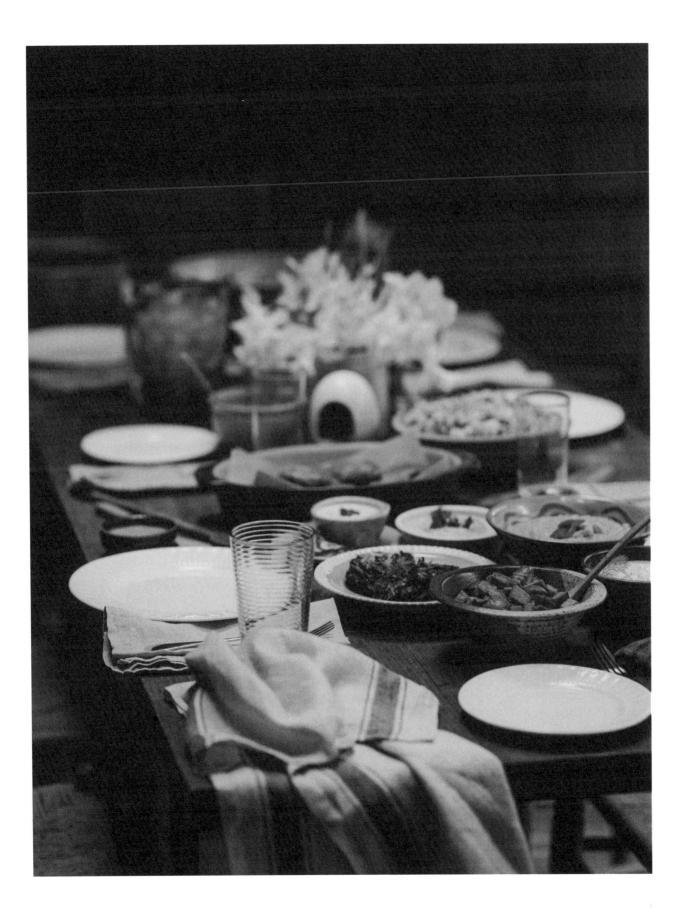

This is a family original, written when our firstborn started to eat meals with us at the table. We wanted to create a practice of thankfulness for the gift it is that we're able to have enough food to enjoy and nourish us and remind ourselves of all the different people involved with the process of the food traveling from the farm to our plates.

—*Jaynie*

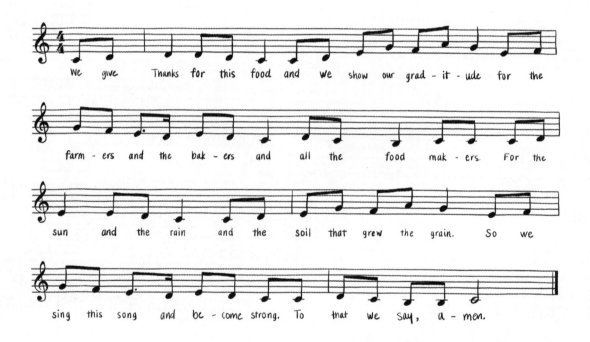

We give Thanks for this food and we show our grad - it - ude for the farm - ers and the bak - ers and all the food mak - ers. For the sun and the rain and the soil that grew the grain. So we sing this song and be - come strong. To that we say, a - men.

This is a traditional children's grace, a well-known prayer recited at mealtimes. We learned it in song form, passed down to us from the older generation at our church who had learned it as children from their parents. Potluck meals at our church often begin with singing this prayer. These words have been put to many different tunes. Around our dinner table we sing it to the tune of "Take My Life and Let It Be."

—*Heather*

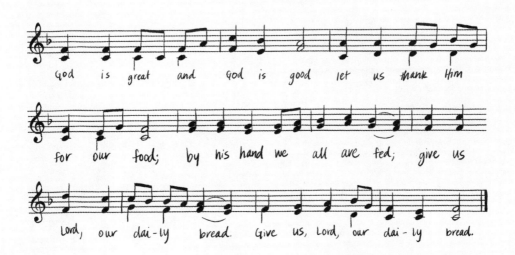

God is great and God is good let us thank Him

for our food; by his hand we all are fed; give us

Lord, our dai-ly bread. Give us, Lord, our dai-ly bread.

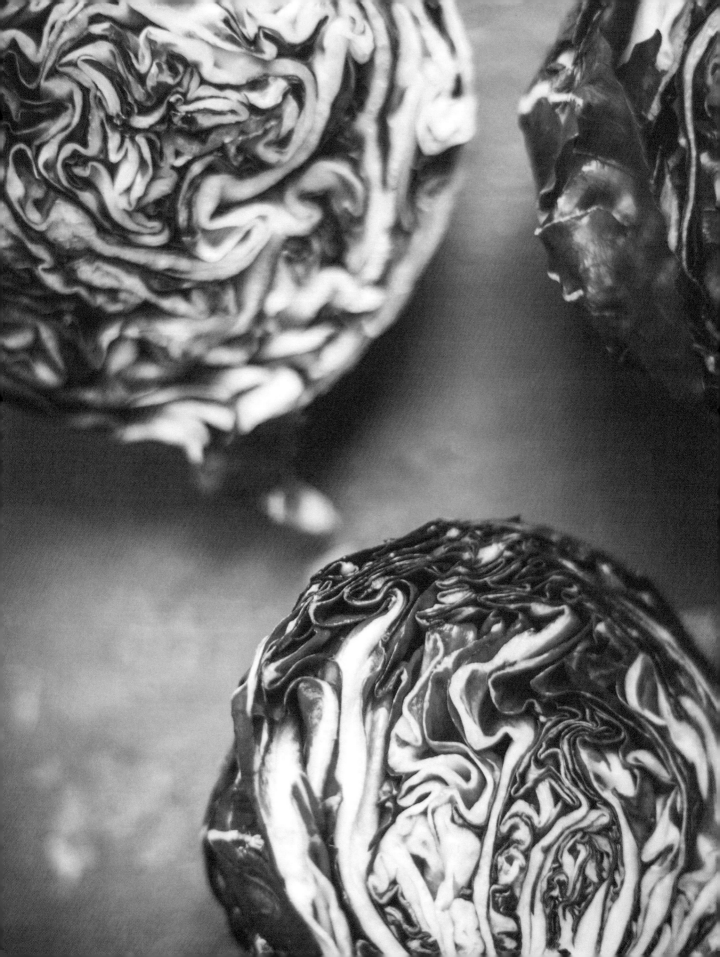

NOTHING WILL BENEFIT HUMAN HEALTH
AND INCREASE CHANCES FOR SURVIVAL
OF LIFE ON EARTH AS MUCH AS THE
EVOLUTION TO A VEGETARIAN DIET.

attributed to Albert Einstein

Planet

Reports about Earth's health are grim. The five years between 2014 and 2018 were the hottest on record, with seventeen of the eighteen warmest years on record occurring since 2001.[7] Ice caps are melting. Sea levels are rising. Storms are getting stronger and more unpredictable. Plastic is polluting our oceans. Invasive species are increasing threats. We are on the brink of the sixth mass extinction, if it isn't already underway. Biodiversity is being lost at unprecedented rates.

What are we to do? Let's go back to the beginning—the beginning when God created everything, proclaimed it good, and gave us the gift of food and the responsibility of stewarding Earth. Eating is an environmental act, with every food choice affecting the world around us. These days most of us no longer till our own soil. To be good stewards, to be informed consumers and responsible eaters, to reconnect with the food we eat, and to work toward right relationship with our planet, we need to ask questions:

- What is the ecological footprint of my food—that is, how much feed, water, land, and fossil fuel energy were consumed? How many emissions were created?

- How far did that food travel to get to my plate? Was it from a local farm or flown in from another country?

- Was my food grown or raised in a way that protected water and soil? Or were contaminating chemical fertilizers used? Was soil health nurtured by thoughtful crop rotating, or was it depleted and then injected with chemical fertilizers?

- Did agricultural practices promote biodiversity? Or were monocrops (when the same crop is grown year after year on the same land) planted and then sprayed with pesticides and herbicides?

- How much packaging waste does my diet generate? How much food do I throw away?

There is a lot to think about in terms of sustainability as it relates to diet. Considering the ecological footprint tied to the production of foods helps guide more eco-friendly eating. Beef, lamb, and goat have by far the largest footprint. Then come cheese, pork, and poultry in the rankings. By comparison, plant proteins, such as whole grains, beans, and lentils, have very small footprints. Ounce per ounce, lentils and meat have roughly the same amount of protein (seven grams per ounce), yet the carbon emissions associated with beef are estimated to be more than twenty-seven times higher than those for lentils.[8] That means vastly different environmental impacts for a similar nutrient value.

Continuing to consume animal proteins at our current rate is unsustainable. USDA data for 2018 reports consumption (called "disappearance") of red meat and poultry by Americans at 219.9 pounds per person each year.[9] In rankings of the top meat-eating countries, the United States is second only to Australia.[10] We cannot keep eating this much meat and expect Earth's resources to be able to regenerate.

But eco-friendly eating is so much more than just animal products versus plants. The story of how any food was grown or raised, processed, and transported matters—a lot. Grass-fed beef from a diversified local farm will have a significantly smaller footprint than beef imported from a large-scale industrialized farm—whether organic or conventional—that is a confined animal feeding operation (CAFO). Dry beans bought in bulk are a significantly more sustainable choice than refrigerated, plastic-packaged tofu processed from genetically modified soybeans, grown as monocrops on huge industrialized farms with gas-guzzling machinery and regular application of chemical fertilizers. Our food system is heavily dependent on fossil fuels, but thoughtful choices can lessen that dependence.

According to the Intergovernmental Panel on Climate Change, the sector of agriculture, forestry, and other land uses accounts for more global emissions than the entire transportation sector.[11] Unsustainable industrialized agricultural practices, highly reliant on fossil fuels, make food one of the largest contributors to our personal carbon footprint. From farm to table, reform is required.

Addressing food and packaging waste is paramount. In a report entitled Wasted, the Natural Resources Defense Council cites that an estimated 40 percent of all food produced in the United States is thrown out.[12] While composting is gaining traction in America, food remains the category of material solid waste with the highest landfill rate, with 76 percent of food scraps generated ending up at the landfill. Twenty-two percent of total landfill weight is from food waste. When organic matter such as rotting food breaks down in the landfill, it releases methane, a potent greenhouse gas estimated to be 25 percent more powerful than CO_2 when it comes to global warming. And this is in addition to the resources consumed by having to grow more food. Food waste happens at every step along the way from farm to table—imperfect produce gets removed by farmers and stores before ever reaching a consumer. Reducing food waste at home begins with good meal planning (see meal planning section on p. 295). Containers and packaging—much of it from food—make up the majority of waste generated in America. Despite a relatively high rate of recycling, 53 percent, for this category of material solid waste, that still leaves containers and packaging accounting for 21 percent of total landfill weight.[13] If you look at what is littering the sides of roads, beaches, and waterways, you will notice it is predominantly food packaging. What are we to do about all this waste? Refuse. Reduce. Repurpose. Reuse. Recycle. Rot (compost). As we become more informed about our food, our complacency is challenged and we are compelled to action.

The recipes in this cookbook are designed to be eco-friendly. The most obvious way we've designed this book to be eco-friendly is in promoting a plant-based diet. All our recipes are vegetarian. Many are vegan. A 2019 report from thirty leading scientists summed up the science this way: "Many studies have assessed environmental effects of various diets, with most finding decreasing effects with increased replacement of animal source foods with plant-based foods. Vegan and vegetarian diets were associated with the greatest reductions in greenhouse-gas emissions and land use."[14]

Within individual recipes and the collection as a whole, we promote diversity in foods. We try to build in flexibility with ingredients, inviting you to substitute what you have on hand or what you or your household prefers. We all have our favorites, but we also invite you to explore lesser-known or unfamiliar ingredients. Trying new things will be increasingly important as the climate changes

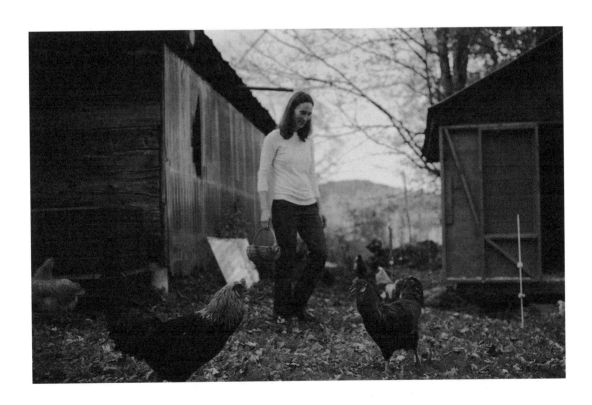

and types of crops (and our tastes) must be adapted to what can be grown.

We make a concerted effort to minimize food waste. We don't have you peel most fruits or vegetables. We find ways to use all edible parts such as carrot or beet tops, squash seeds and skins, and broccoli stems. (Bonus: you get nutritional benefits from these things.) By-products such as whey and buttermilk are incorporated into other recipes. And the liquid saved from cooking beans or drained from a can of beans, called aquafaba, is often incorporated into our recipes.

Packaging waste is also kept to a minimum. We invite you to cook—a lot. Cooking more means relying less on packaged, processed foods. We invite you to make your own foods whenever possible, providing recipes for ingredients that would otherwise come in containers, such as nut butters, tortillas, yogurt, broth, butter, canned tomatoes, and pasta.

We have given thought to energy consumption in the kitchen and discovered that preheating your oven is unnecessary (unless baking with leaveners). By questioning common cooking techniques, we realized that we often do things in the kitchen simply because we were taught or told a particular way is best. Another way we conserve energy is through the practice of seasonal eating

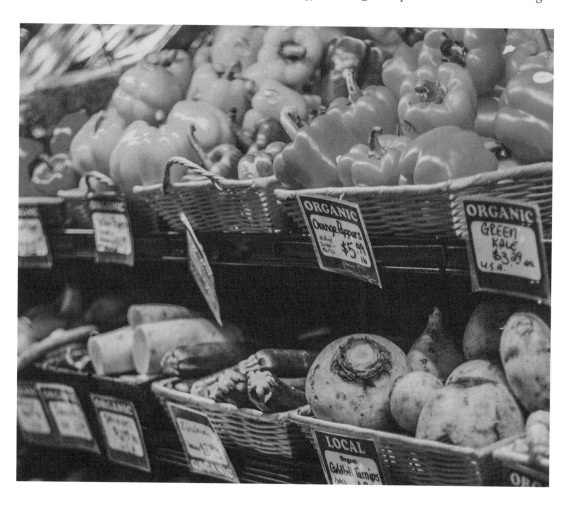

and the use of local foods. You will find recipes for all seasons—recipes that make use of what is growing in the garden and locally available. We'll even teach you how to preserve the harvest by canning. As less food is transported, fewer emissions are generated.

We encourage you to use food dollars in support of healthy agricultural practices that support healthy ecosystems. Here are some ideas.

Buy organic. By definition, organic foods are those grown without the use of synthetic fertilizers, herbicides, or pesticides and that are non-GMO (genetically modified organism). Organic farming practices must promote ecological balance, conserve biodiversity, and cycle resources. That said, foods lacking an organic label are not necessarily grown unsustainably. There is a cost for growers to become organically certified, and some choose not to go through that intensive and financially burdensome process. And just because something is labeled organic doesn't automatically make it the best choice. For example, organic, cage-free eggs may still be factory-farmed, with chickens living in appalling conditions.

Organic foods usually cost more, so if you can't buy everything organic, you can focus on some foods. The Environmental Working Group annually publishes a list called "The Dirty Dozen" and "The Clean Fifteen," ranking produce they find to have the highest and lowest levels of pesticide residue. Regularly consumed GMO crops that were engineered to be herbicide resistant, such as soy, corn, canola, and sugar beets, can be another place where food dollars are well spent on organic over conventional.

Buy local. When buying local, you can talk to the grower, visit the farm, get to know how your food is grown, and feel confident in your source even if it has not been certified organic. Those benefits are all in addition to the energy savings that come from not transporting food long distances. Look for local foods at your grocery store, visit a farmers' market or farmer's stand, or join a CSA (community-supported agriculture), in which you buy a share of produce at the beginning of the season, thereby sharing some of the risk with the farmer and regularly receiving a box of locally grown produce.

Plant a garden. A backyard garden is another example of sourcing local—hyperlocal! This connects you most directly to your food, allowing you to be present from planting to plating.

We know an environmental crisis is before us. So how should we live and how should we cook now? When we look at massive environmental problems, we may be tempted to conclude that personal small effort won't make much difference. Resist and reject that mentality. Diet is a powerful driver of environmental issues. Since we all need to eat, we all have an opportunity to consume less meat and fewer dairy products and to throw away less food. We can all eat more locally sourced, minimally packaged, sustainably produced, seasonal, plant-based food. Together, we can become faithful stewards of Earth.

Sustainability Steps

Planet-conscious food choices don't happen all at once. Give yourself some grace as you start this journey. Take steps toward sustainability, and enjoy learning as you go!

START SMALL

- Eat more meatless meals
- Choose seasonal foods
- Buy organic and local
- Bring your own (BYO) bags to shop

KEEP GOING

- Eat predominantly a plant-based diet
- Join a food co-op
- Purchase a CSA share
- Compost (see technique on p. 308)

GO FURTHER

- Eat exclusively a plant-based diet
- Garden organically
- Make your own staples
- Can, dry, and freeze to preserve the harvest
- Use all edible parts of food
- Buy in bulk using BYO containers
- Avoid foods in plastic packaging
- Go wildcrafting with care

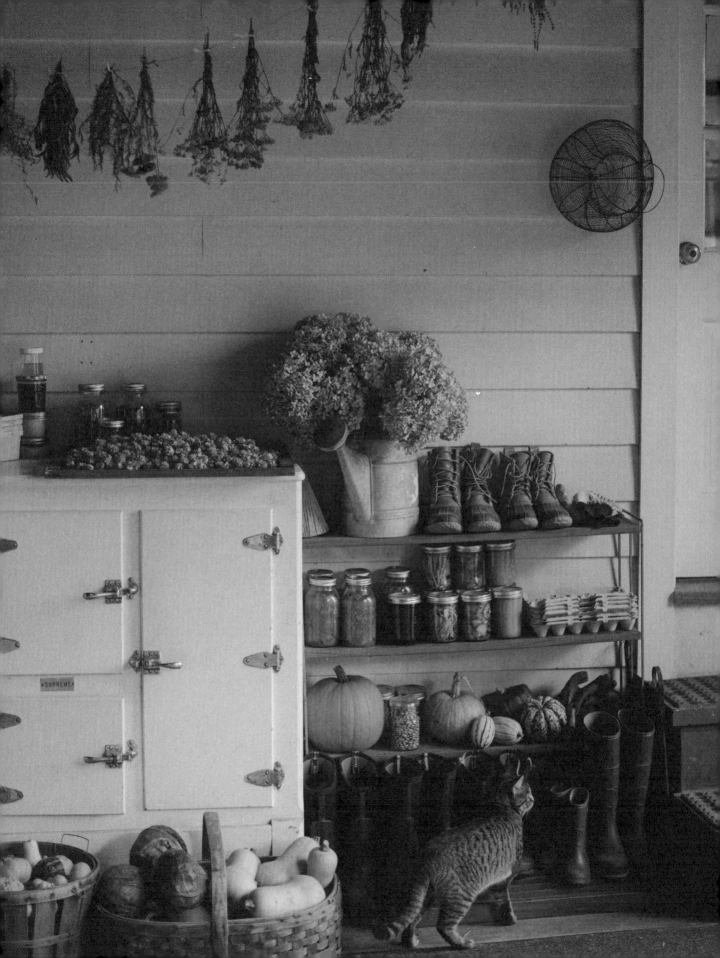

ORGANIC
LACINATO
$3.39 ea
U.S.A

ORGANIC
Dandelion Greens
$2.99 each

COKE
FARM
Organic
Green Dandelion
PLU #

ORGANIC
ALL LETTUCE
$3.49 EA.
U.S.A.

Nutrition 101

Our bodies use food for fuel. Calories—the amount of energy contained in a food—come from carbohydrates, fats, and proteins. We require a mix of all three. General dietary guidance is for total daily calories to be 45–65 percent carbohydrate, 20–35 percent fat, and 10–35 percent protein. For best health, quality counts when making choices in each category.

Carbohydrates

Dietary recommendations are for about half of total calories to come from carbohydrates. This makes sense when you count up how many food groups contain carbs: fruits, vegetables, grains, and dairy. Carbohydrates are the primary and preferred fuel for our brain and muscles. In recent years many fad diets have focused on limiting carbohydrates. In part, this trend is in response to the overabundance of processed, unhealthy carbohydrate products available. When we refocus on healthy eating, we are intentional about choosing carbohydrates in their whole form. Berries. Beans. Barley. Healthy, unprocessed, plant-based, carbohydrate-rich foods include:

WHOLE GRAINS: Dietary guidelines for Americans advise that at least half the grains we eat each day should be whole grains. In this cookbook we use 100 percent whole grains almost 100 percent of the time.

NATURAL SUGARS: Fructose (fruit sugar) and lactose (milk sugar) are carbohydrates that occur naturally in nutrient-rich fruits and dairy. Enjoy them. Fruits and dairy are the basis of many of our desserts, making use of this natural sweetness.

FIBER: Whole grains, fruits, vegetables (which include legumes), and nuts and seeds all contain fiber, an indigestible carbohydrate. Fiber helps us to feel full, aids bowel regularity, lowers cholesterol, regulates blood sugar, and is associated with protection against many diseases. These alone are excellent reasons to eat a plant-based diet. One caveat: If you are not used to eating fiber, add it gradually into your diet and increase the amount of fluid you drink. This will help your digestive system adapt while limiting possible discomfort from gas and bloating.

Fats

Fats help us to feel full, and they play important roles in our bodies, such as the absorption of fat-soluble vitamins and the production of hormones. In general, healthy fats come from plants and fish, while unhealthy fats are human-made and from animals.

TRANS FATS: These predominantly human-made fats proved especially unhealthy and were banned from the food supply in 2018. Good riddance!

SATURATED FATS: Limit intake of unhealthy saturated fats, which come from animal sources (such as red meat, poultry skin, dairy fat) and tropical oils (such as palm and coconut). In this cookbook we let you decide what fat-content milk or yogurt you wish to use in recipes (ranging from fat-free skim to whole 3.5 percent), but we advise you to use these in moderation.

UNSATURATED FATS: Healthy fats from plants! Monounsaturated fats (such as olive and canola oil) are considered to be the best choices. Polyunsaturated fats (such as vegetable, sunflower, safflower, and avocado oil) are good choices. In our recipes we liberally use healthy unsaturated fats in the form of oils, nuts, seeds, and avocados. Our go-tos for most recipes are the monounsaturated options: olive oil for flavor and organic canola oil (which also contains omega-3) for a neutral choice.

OMEGA-3: An essential fat that our body cannot make; we must obtain it through diet. Fish is considered the best source of omega-3. Some pescatarians who otherwise maintain a vegetarian diet elect to eat fish for this very reason. Since we do not include fish in this cookbook (fish is technically defined as meat since it is the flesh of an animal), we look to plant-based sources of omega-3. Canola oil, walnuts, and flaxseed are some of these sources.

Proteins

Most Americans get far too much. Protein is found in many foods, including vegetables and whole grains. Protein-rich nuts, seeds, dry beans, lentils, eggs, and dairy are also good sources.

QUALITY: Animal proteins are considered "complete," containing all essential amino acids. Most plant proteins are incomplete. Different plant proteins have different amino acid mixes. Diets that include a variety of foods will get a sufficient mix of amino acids, the building blocks of protein, that your body needs. There is no need to combine specific foods on the basis of their amino acid profiles, such as rice with beans, at a single meal in order to create a complete protein.

SOY: A complete plant protein (that is, containing all the essential amino acids), soy is a high-quality nutritional choice and encouraged in a healthy diet. Concerns about estrogenic effects of soy foods are unfounded. Because soy is often a GMO crop, sourcing organically may be desirable on the basis of environmental concerns. We include soy foods such as edamame (green, immature soybean), tempeh, and tofu.

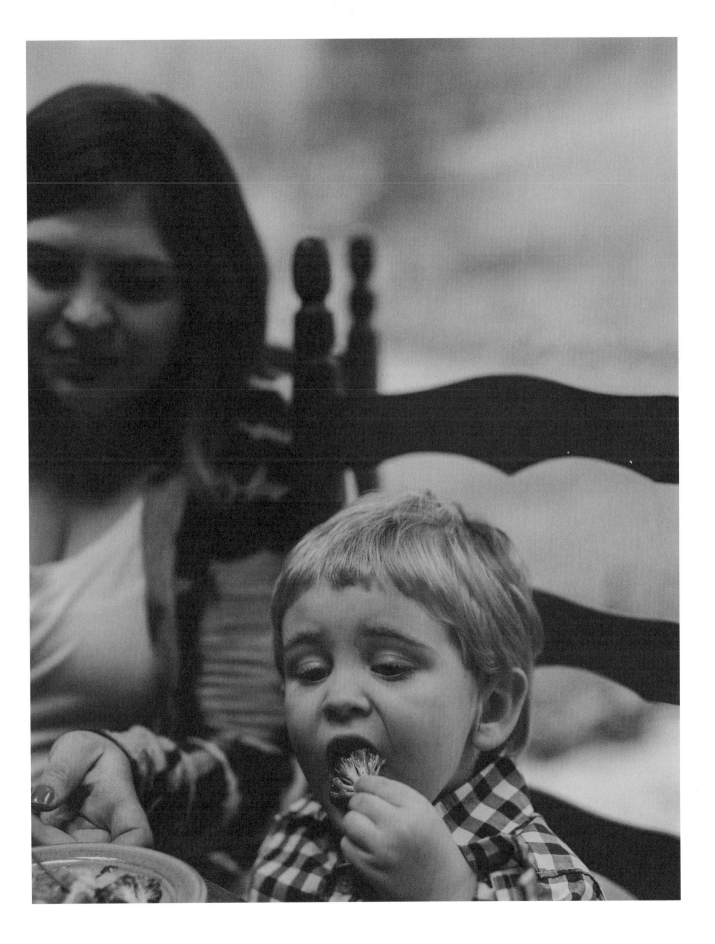

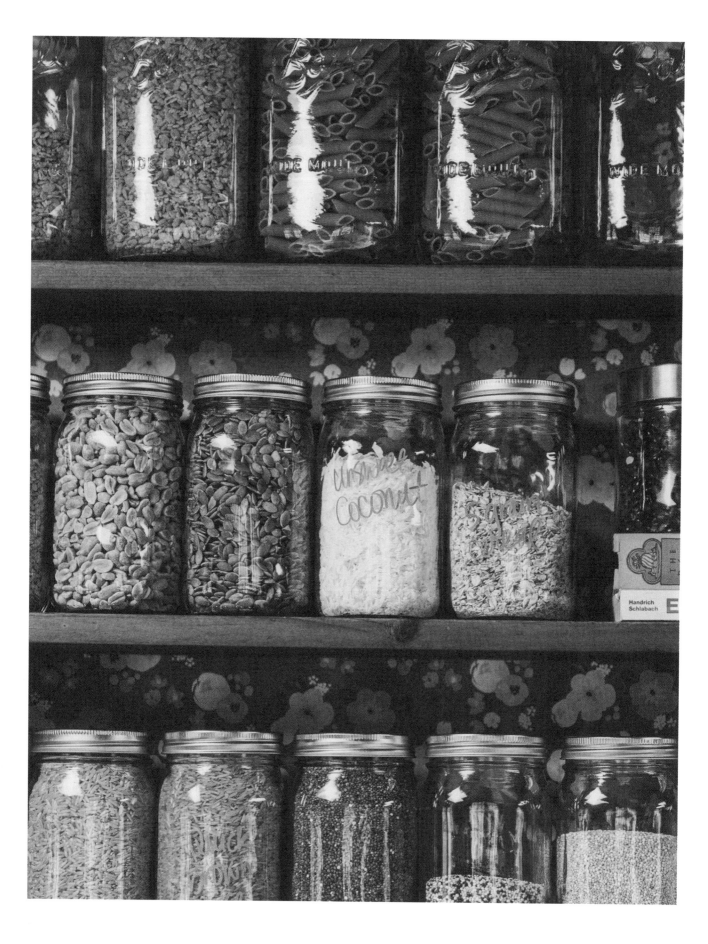

A Well-Stocked Kitchen

The best way to ensure success in cooking at home regularly is to keep your kitchen well stocked with the essentials. It's also key to saving you time and money. Below are things we always have on hand that get used regularly. These items are also great for substituting when another ingredient, less often used but similar, might be called for in a recipe.

Sustainable staples

Have these foods on hand, and you will be well prepared to make many of our recipes.

WHOLE GRAINS

Grains in their whole form retain all nutritional goodness from bran, germ, and endosperm. Bran is the outer fiber-containing shell. Germ is the nutrient-rich core. Endosperm is the starchy inside, the only component that remains when you refine a grain. Whole grains are an excellent source of healthy carbohydrates, dietary fiber, and nutrients. They also contain some healthy fats that can go rancid over time, so store whole grain flour in your refrigerator or freezer for optimal freshness. Bob's Red Mill and King Arthur Flour are two great sources for whole grain products.

BROWN RICE	WHEAT BERRIES	QUINOA
WHOLE WHEAT COUSCOUS	ROLLED OATS	WHOLE WHEAT FLOUR

VEGETABLES

These sturdy vegetables—fresh, canned, and frozen—are the basis for many meals. Supplement with more perishable or recipe-specific ones when called for.

GARLIC	CARROTS	SWEET POTATOES
ONIONS	CELERY	FROZEN CORN, PEAS, EDAMAME, AND SPINACH
SHALLOTS	CANNED DICED TOMATOES	

FRUITS

These fresh, dried, and frozen fruits are go-tos that don't go bad quickly. Supplement with more perishable or recipe-specific ones when called for.

APPLES	LIMES	DRIED CRANBERRIES
LEMONS	RAISINS	FROZEN BERRIES

PROTEINS

Plant-based protein foods include pulses (edible seeds of plants in the legume family, including beans, dry peas, and lentils), soy-based foods, nuts, and seeds. Eggs and dairy are also rich proteins sourced from animals.

BEANS: DRY AND/OR CANNED (FOR QUICK MEALS)	TOFU (FIRM OR EXTRA FIRM)	EGGS
	NUTS AND NUT BUTTER (REFRIGERATE FOR BEST FRESHNESS)	MILK
PEAS		PLAIN GREEK YOGURT
LENTILS	SEEDS AND SEED BUTTERS	HARD CHEESE

OILS

If we could have just two cooking oils, they would be olive oil and organic canola oil. Both are high in heart-healthy monounsaturated fats. Olive oil imparts flavor to food, while canola is considered a neutral oil. There are two types of olive oil. Refined olive oil has a lighter flavor and higher smoke point and is a good choice for all-purpose cooking. Extra-virgin olive oil has a robust flavor and lower smoke point, making it best for vinaigrettes or as a finishing oil drizzled on top of a soup or mixed into a dip.

Canola oil endears itself to us because it is a source of omega-3 fatty acids, an essential fat that our bodies need. Concerns about toxins in canola are unfounded; however, most conventional canola plant (rapeseed) crops grown are genetically modified to be resistant to herbicides and the oil is often extracted using hexane. Therefore organic may be a preferred choice on the basis of environmental concerns.

There are many other choices for neutral oils; such as safflower oil, sunflower oil, and grapeseed oil. Each will have its own characteristics and a different mix of fatty acids. There is health in diversity. Spend some time exploring the options and choose the ones you want to have on hand. Do not keep too many on hand at any given time, however, as oils do go rancid over time. For optimal freshness, store oils away from heat (not next to your stove) and away from light (in dark bottles, in a pantry).

REGULAR (LIGHT) OLIVE OIL	EXTRA-VIRGIN OLIVE OIL	AVOCADO OIL
CANOLA OIL	TOASTED SESAME OIL	GRAPESEED OIL

Ingredients that add taste and contribute to aroma of food, these flavorings play very important supporting roles in recipes. To keep sodium in check, choose reduced sodium versions of broth and soy sauce.

VEGETABLE BROTH	NUTRITIONAL YEAST	VERMOUTH (SHELF-STABLE SUBSTITUTE FOR WHITE WINE)
SOY SAUCE OR TAMARI	DIJON MUSTARD	

HERBS (DRIED)

OREGANO	PARSLEY	DILL WEED
BASIL	THYME	BAY LEAVES

SPICES

GROUND CUMIN	CURRY POWDER (SPICE BLEND)	HOT RED PEPPER FLAKES
CHILI POWDER (SPICE BLEND)		PAPRIKA
	BLACK PEPPER	CINNAMON

SALTS

KOSHER SALT (FOR COOKING)	TABLE SALT (FOR BAKING)	FLAKY SEA SALT (FOR FINISHING)

VINEGARS

BALSAMIC VINEGAR	APPLE CIDER VINEGAR	RED/WHITE WINE VINEGAR

NATURAL SWEETENERS

HONEY	MAPLE SYRUP	DATES

Equipment essentials

These are tools we find most helpful to have in the kitchen.

CUTLERY

Three good knives are all you need, so buy quality ones and keep them honed and sharp. This will make cutting easier, safer, and more enjoyable. Have the knives sharpened as needed, several times per year typically, to restore dulled blades. Maintain your sharp knives by honing the chef and paring knives each time you use them, or more often during a big chopping job. Honing straightens out the blade's edge, which can get out of alignment during use.

CHEF'S KNIFE (8-INCH; A SECOND 6-INCH, ESPECIALLY FOR SMALLER HANDS)	PARING KNIFE	HONING STEEL
	BREAD KNIFE	CUTTING BOARDS

POWERED TOOLS

If we could only have one powered tool, it would be the food processor. This workhorse makes quick work of chopping, shredding, and pureeing. Many of our make-your-own recipes require this tool. The other items listed are nice but not necessary. If you don't have a food processor, a high-powered blender can work for many of the pureed foods. When pureeing hot items, an immersion blender eliminates the need to transfer hot liquids. A multicooker can be a big time-saver: its pressure-cook function can decrease cook time for dry beans and whole grains almost by half, and the slow-cook function is great for set-it-and-forget-it meals. Having a spice grinder guarantees freshness when our recipes call for freshly ground flaxseed or black pepper. If you frequently make doughs such as bread, pizza, or pasta, machines are worthwhile investments.

FOOD PROCESSOR	IMMERSION BLENDER	MULTICOOKER (SLOW COOKER, PRESSURE COOKER, RICE COOKER COMBINED)
BLENDER	SPICE GRINDER OR MILL	

POTS AND PANS

There are just a few essentials, so once again buy quality items that will last. Fully clad stainless steel and cast iron are a cook's best choices.

LARGE DUTCH OVEN OR HEAVY-BOTTOMED POT WITH LID	STAINLESS STEEL:
LARGE AND MEDIUM CAST-IRON SKILLETS	SAUCEPANS WITH LIDS, SMALL, MEDIUM, AND LARGE
GRIDDLE (SPANNING TWO BURNERS; CAST IRON IS NICE)	LARGE SKILLET WITH LID

Type of material and color will affect how recipes come out. Dark-colored bakeware will absorb and reflect more heat and is desirable for roasting and browning. In this cookbook we tested recipes in metal bakeware (except for casserole items, which were tested in either glass or ceramic). We use dark-colored baking sheets for roasting. If you have light-colored baking sheets, you should adjust the recipe to increase oven temperature by 25°F or lengthen time by about 5 minutes. If you use glass baking dishes, lower the oven temperature by 25°F and bake up to 10 minutes longer.

BAKING SHEETS (ALSO KNOWN AS SHEET PANS)	BAKING PANS (9 X 13-INCH AND 8 X 8-INCH)	PIE DISH
		MUFFIN TINS

HAND TOOLS

BOX GRATER	LEMON AND LIME SQUEEZER/ JUICER	8-OUNCE JAR WITH TIGHT-FITTING LID (TO SHAKE SALAD DRESSINGS)
CAN OPENER		
COLANDER	MANDOLINE (FOR FAST, EVEN THICKNESS IN SLICING)	EXTRA ICE CUBE TRAY (FOR FREEZING INDIVIDUAL SERVINGS OF PESTO, CHIPOTLE PEPPERS, MASALA PASTE, COMPOTE)
FINE-MESH SIEVE		
FOOD MILL (TO SEPARATE SEEDS AND SKINS TO MAKE A PUREE, LIKE TOMATO OR APPLE SAUCE)	MICROPLANE GRATER	
	PASTA FORK	TORTILLA PRESS (IF MAKING TORTILLAS OFTEN)
	POTATO MASHER, PASTRY CUTTER	
GARLIC PRESS	VEGETABLE PEELER	SALAD SPINNER

MIX AND MEASURE

MIXING SPOONS	SPATULA	GLASS LIQUID MEASURING CUPS
SLOTTED SPOON	MEASURING CUPS	
SOUP LADLE	MEASURING SPOONS	MIXING BOWLS (SMALL, MEDIUM, LARGE)
WHISK	KITCHEN SCALE (FOR BAKING)	

FOOD STORAGE

When it comes to food packaging, plastic is pervasive. In a sustainable kitchen we want to limit use of plastic, especially single-use products. Thankfully, there are good alternatives available.

- beeswax wraps (a reusable and compostable alternative to plastic wrap)

- silicone or cotton bowl and dish covers (or our favorite: simply put a plate over your bowl!)

- reusable produce bags (for grocery shopping; keep with your reusable shopping bags, ready to go)

- reusable sandwich/snack wraps or bags (made from beeswax, cotton, paper, or silicone)

- glass or stainless steel containers with lids (for leftovers)

- glass containers with lids, such as quart canning jars (for bulk dry goods; keep with your reusable shopping/produce bags)

- silicone food bags (for freezing)

- compostable parchment paper (reuse if possible)

- 100 percent recycled aluminum foil (reuse if possible)

- flour sack cloths (very versatile and a reusable alternative to paper towels and cheesecloth: keep a stack on hand for pressing tofu; covering dough during proofing; drying produce, dishes, and hands)

- kitchen compost pail (for food scraps)

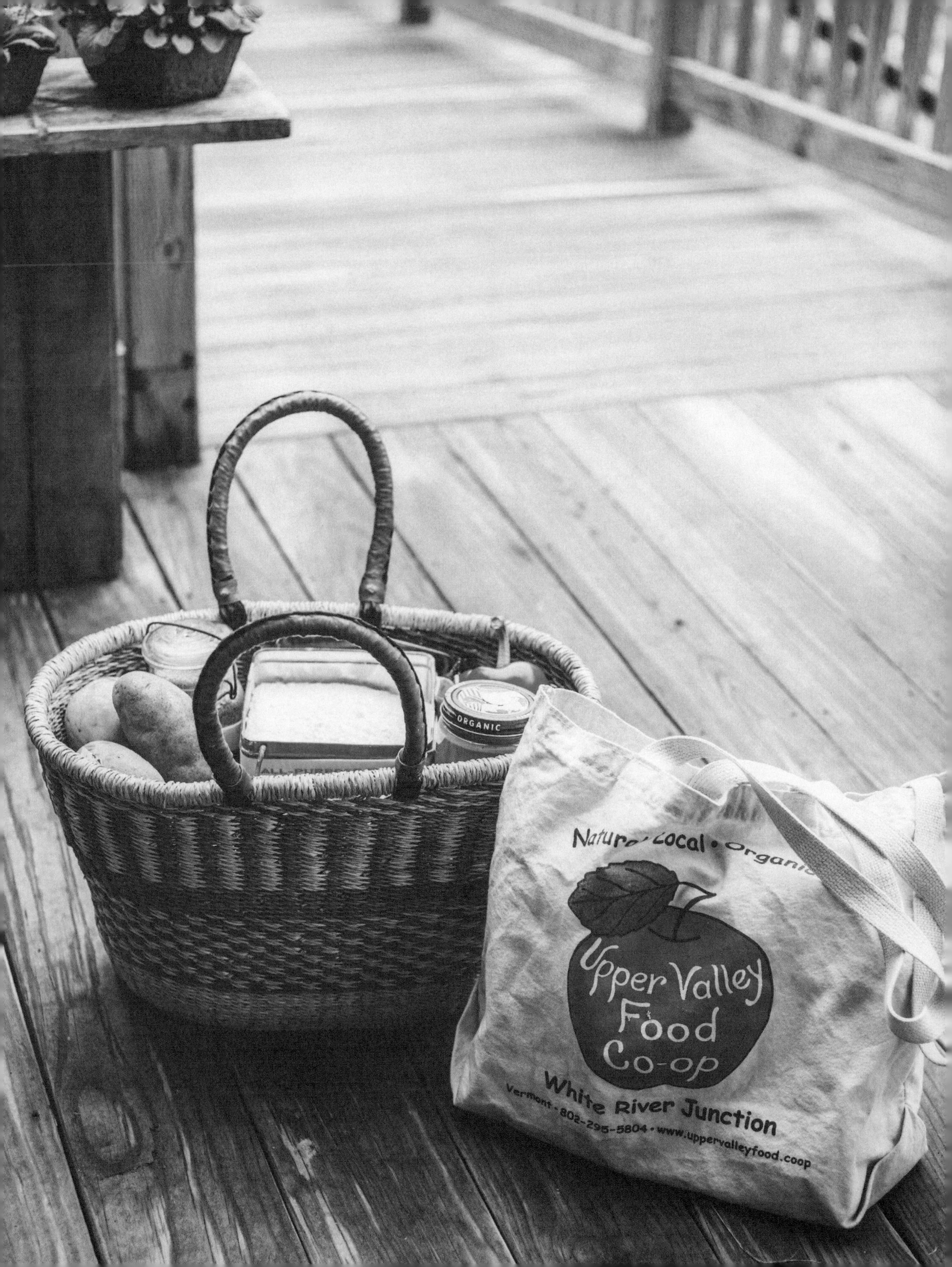
ORGANIC
Upper Valley Food Co-op
White River Junction
Vermont • 802-295-5804 • www.uppervalleyfood.coop

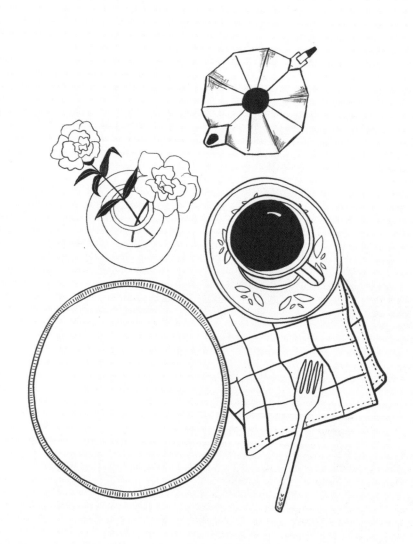

Breakfasts

———

Veggie-Studded Frittata

A frittata comes together more quickly than a quiche and saves a lot of unhealthy, saturated fat calories by not having a crust or cream. Vegetables that work well in this dish include bell pepper, mushroom, zucchini, and broccoli. Serve with a whole grain on the side to complete the meal.

SERVES 4

7 eggs

½ teaspoon kosher salt

¼ teaspoon freshly ground black pepper

2 tablespoons olive oil

½ cup chopped onion

2½ cups chopped vegetables (one kind or a medley)

4 ounces cheddar cheese, shredded (about 1 cup)

Whisk together eggs, salt, and pepper. Set aside.

Heat oil in a large oven-safe skillet (such as cast iron or all stainless steel) over medium heat. Add onion. Sauté for 5 minutes, or until onions begin to soften. Add remaining vegetables. Sauté for another 5 minutes, or until tender.

Pour egg mixture over vegetables in the skillet. Cook until eggs are almost set. It can help to run a heatproof spatula around the edges, tipping the skillet slightly, to let uncooked egg from the center drain over to the edges, where it'll cook more quickly.

Sprinkle cheese over the top. Place skillet in a cold oven on the top rack closest to the broiler. Turn broiler on high. Cook until eggs are set and cheese is beginning to brown, about 3 minutes (watch closely so as not to burn). Cool slightly before serving.

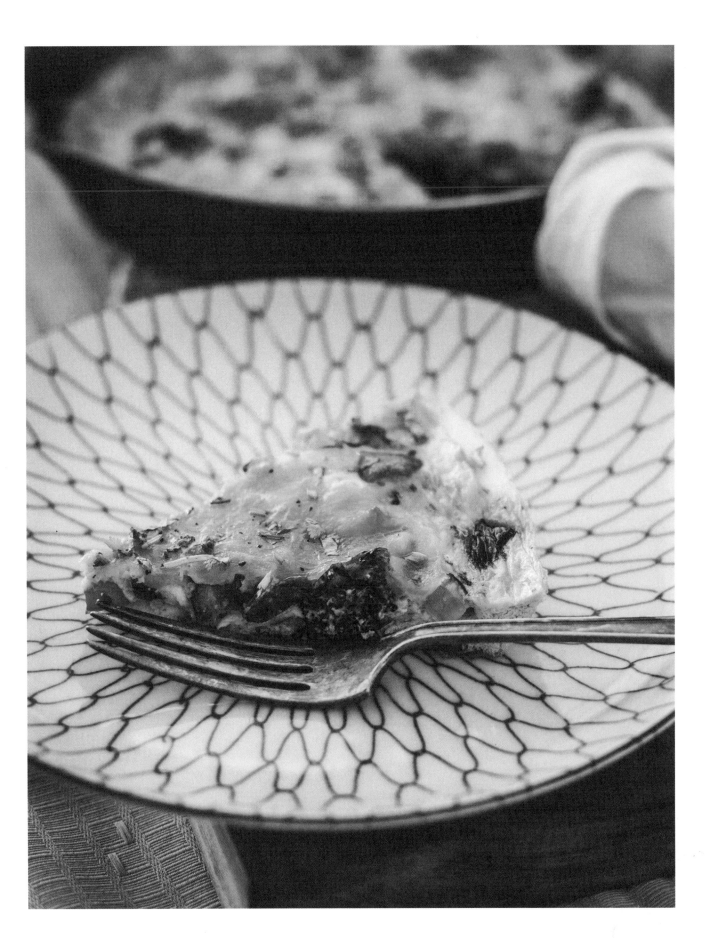

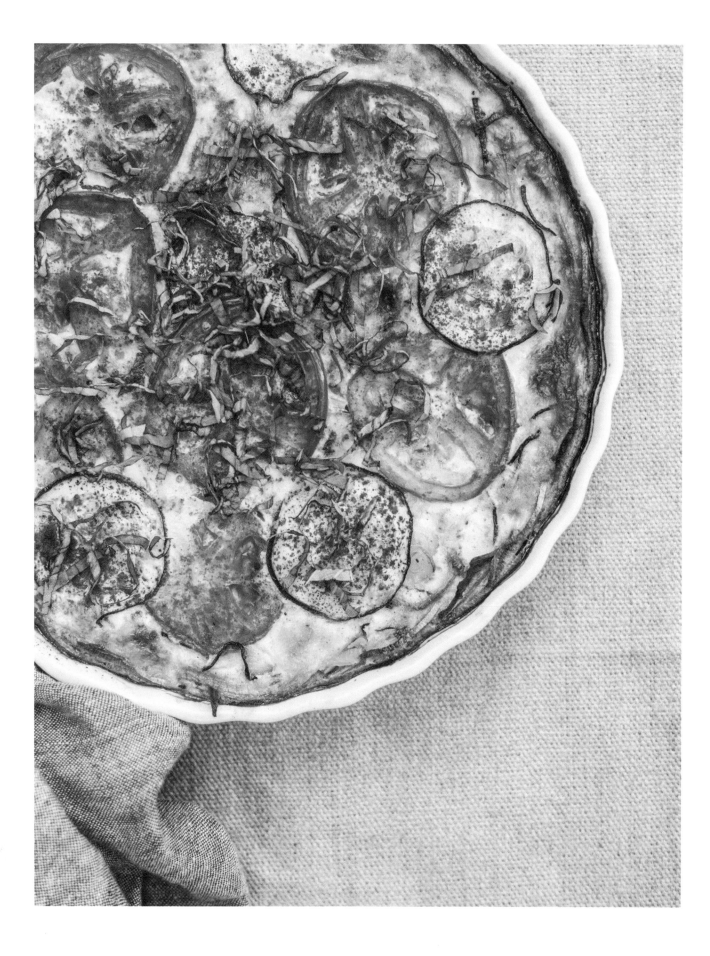

End-of-Summer Quiche

When zucchini and tomatoes are everywhere, this is a great way to use them. Just about any veggies you have on hand could appear in this quiche. Just give yourself plenty of cooking and baking time.

SERVES 6

1 large or 2 medium sweet potatoes

3 teaspoons olive oil, divided, plus additional for oiling dish

2 cups sliced zucchini (⅛-inch-thick slices)

½ red onion, thinly sliced

kosher salt and freshly ground black pepper

4 large eggs

1 cup milk

1 tablespoon chopped fresh basil plus additional for garnish

¼ teaspoon dry mustard

¼ teaspoon cayenne, or as desired

4 ounces Gruyère or cheddar cheese, shredded (about 1 cup)

paprika (optional)

1 small tomato, sliced ⅛ inch thick

NOTE: If you have leftover sweet potato slices, toss them with olive oil, salt, and pepper and roast them on a separate baking sheet to nibble on later.

Slice the sweet potatoes into rounds about ¼ inch thick. Lightly oil a pie dish, then fill the bottom of the dish with a layer of sweet potato slices. Cut the remaining sweet potato rounds in half and fill around the edges, rounded side up. Cover dish fully with slices; this may require some overlap, but try to avoid it when possible. Once the dish is filled, drizzle 1 teaspoon oil over the sweet potatoes and gently brush with a basting brush to coat evenly, or use an olive oil spray bottle. Place in a cold oven and turn to 375°F. Start timing and bake for 25 minutes.

While the crust is cooking, heat the remaining 2 teaspoons oil in a large skillet over medium-high heat. Add the zucchini and onion, season with a dash salt and pepper, and cook until lightly browned, about 5 minutes. Set aside.

In a large mixing bowl, whisk the eggs, milk, 1 tablespoon basil, ½ teaspoon salt, ¼ teaspoon pepper, dry mustard, and cayenne. Add cheese to egg mixture along with the cooked vegetables. Stir to combine. Gently pour filling over baked sweet potato crust. Sprinkle with paprika, if desired. Top with a single layer of sliced tomatoes.

Bake for 40–50 minutes, or until egg mixture is set in the center. Cool before serving. Garnish with fresh basil, if desired.

Broccoli Cheddar Crustless Quiche

A full ½ cup serving of broccoli fits easily into each portion thanks to chopping it up finely. A food processor, if you have one, makes quick work of this. Fresh herbs and spices impart flavor.

SERVES 6

1 head broccoli, both stem and florets
(about 1 pound)

4 large eggs

1¼ cups milk

¼ cup finely chopped fresh parsley
plus additional for garnish

2 tablespoons minced fresh chives
plus additional for garnish

¼ teaspoon kosher salt

⅛ teaspoon freshly ground black pepper

⅛ teaspoon ground nutmeg

6 ounces cheddar cheese, shredded
(about 1½ cups)

Prepare broccoli by hand-chopping into individual florets and cutting stems into thin slices. Steam broccoli with a little water until tender but still bright green, either covered in the microwave for about 3 minutes or on the stovetop in a covered saucepan for about 5 minutes.

Use a food processor to chop steamed broccoli into very fine pieces. Do not puree.

Whisk eggs, milk, parsley, chives, salt, pepper, and nutmeg together in a large bowl. Stir the cheddar cheese and broccoli into the egg mixture.

Lightly oil an 8 x 8-inch square baking pan or a 9-inch pie dish. Pour mixture into prepared dish. Place in a cold oven and turn to 375°F. Start timing and bake for about 1 hour, or until egg is set in the middle.

Remove from oven and let sit for about 10 minutes before serving. Garnish with additional chopped parsley, chives, salt, and pepper as desired.

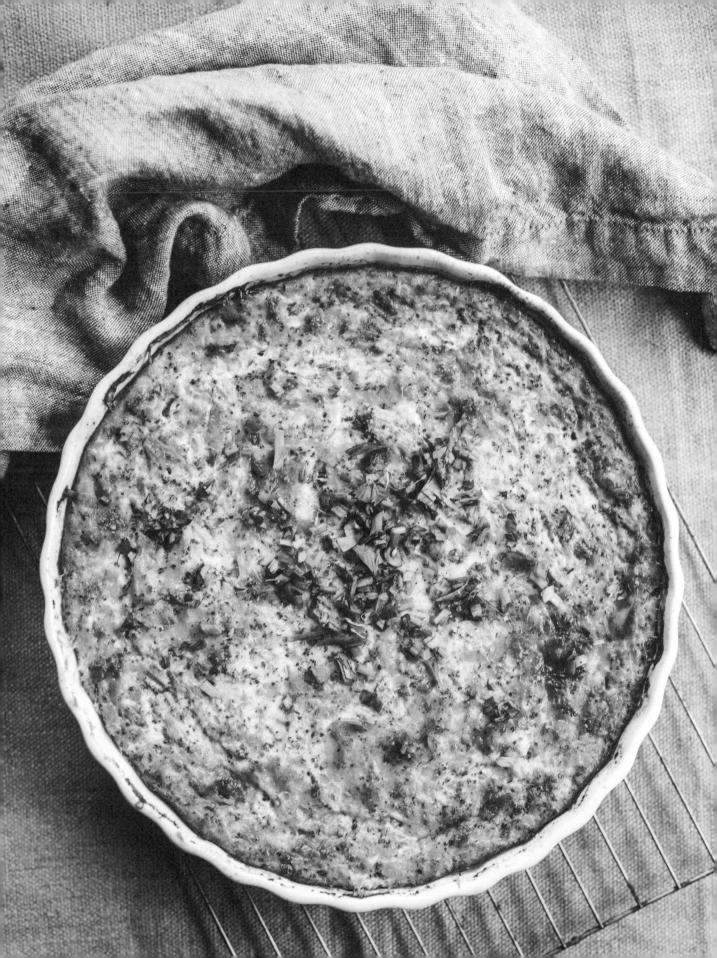

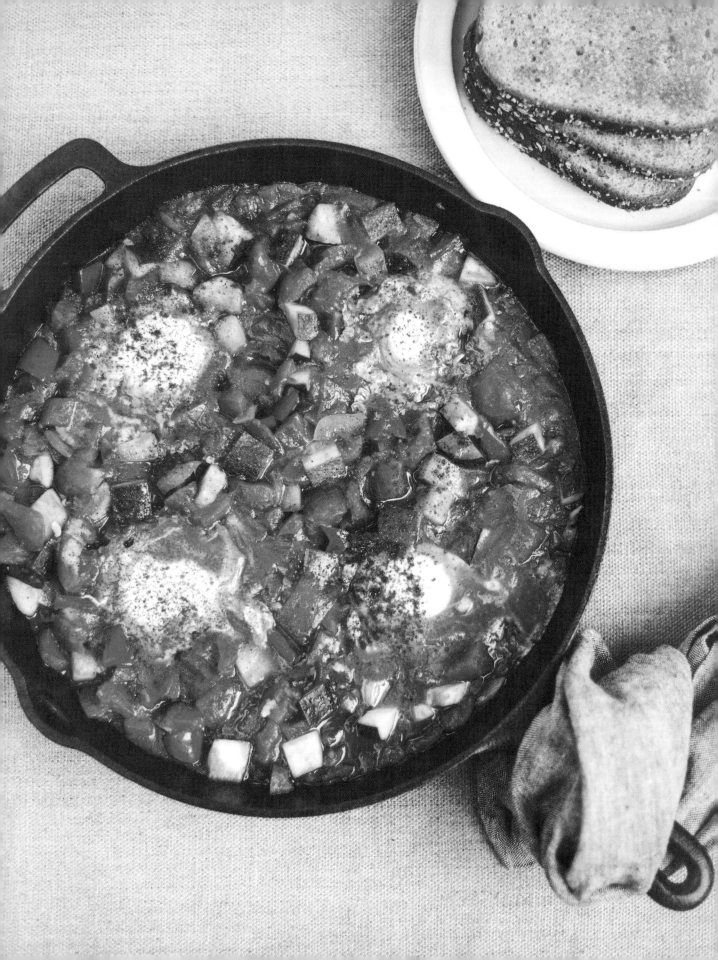

Zucchini Shakshuka

With origins in North Africa along the Mediterranean Sea, shakshuka is a poached egg dish over a savory tomato-vegetable stew. Serve with a side of whole grain toast or over cooked whole wheat couscous.

SERVES 4

3 tablespoons olive oil

1 onion, diced

1 red bell pepper, diced

1 small zucchini, diced

2 cloves garlic, minced

kosher salt

1 teaspoon ground cumin

½ teaspoon hot red pepper flakes (optional)

1 (28-ounce) can diced tomatoes; or 4 cups diced fresh

6 large eggs

dash hot paprika or cayenne (optional)

freshly ground black pepper

In a large skillet with a tight-fitting lid, heat the oil over medium heat.

Add the onion and bell pepper. Stir to coat with the oil. Cover and cook until the onion is softened, 5–7 minutes.

Uncover, stir in the zucchini, garlic, ½ teaspoon salt, cumin, and optional hot red pepper flakes. Cook, uncovered, for 4 minutes, stirring occasionally.

Stir in the tomatoes and simmer until the vegetables are tender, 7–8 minutes.

Use a spoon to make six little wells in the sauce. Working with one egg at time, break an egg into a separate dish, then pour carefully into well in the sauce. Repeat with remaining eggs. Sprinkle the eggs with paprika or cayenne, black pepper, and additional salt, as desired. Cover the skillet and simmer gently until the eggs are poached, 6–8 minutes. Whites will be set at about 6 minutes but yolks will still be runny. For a firmer yolk, cook for a full 7–8 minutes.

MAKE IT YOURSELF

Canned Diced Tomatoes (p. 274)

Breakfast Tacos

Savory wraps that can be enjoyed for breakfast or any meal of the day. For the best scrambled eggs, seek out a local source for your eggs. Go vegan and try these tacos with our Curried Tofu Scramble.

SERVES 4

---

6 eggs; or 1 recipe Curried Tofu Scramble (p. 48)

½ tablespoon oil or melted butter

¼ cup shredded cheddar cheese (optional)

kosher salt and freshly ground black pepper

4 whole wheat tortillas

2 cups Spicy Cauliflower Walnut Chorizo (p. 197)

1 avocado, sliced; or ½ cup Guacamole (p. 257)

Fresh Salsa (p. 254)

If using eggs, scramble eggs: Heat skillet over medium-low or low heat. Coat skillet lightly with oil or melted butter. Whisk eggs well and pour into skillet. Use a spatula to gently fold eggs, pushing them to one side of the skillet and then folding back in, until set but still wet. Eggs may even appear undercooked, but they will continue to cook once removed from heat. It is easy to overcook eggs, which results in them being tough and less tasty. Remove from heat and fold in cheddar cheese, if desired, and season with salt and pepper to taste.

If using Curried Tofu Scramble, it is optional to fold in cheddar cheese once the tofu is warmed. Taste and add more salt and pepper only if desired.

Warm the tortillas if desired.

Down the center of each tortilla, layer scrambled eggs or tofu scramble, chorizo, avocado, and salsa as desired. To eat, roll or fold up.

MAKE IT YOURSELF

Whole Wheat Tortillas (p. 286)

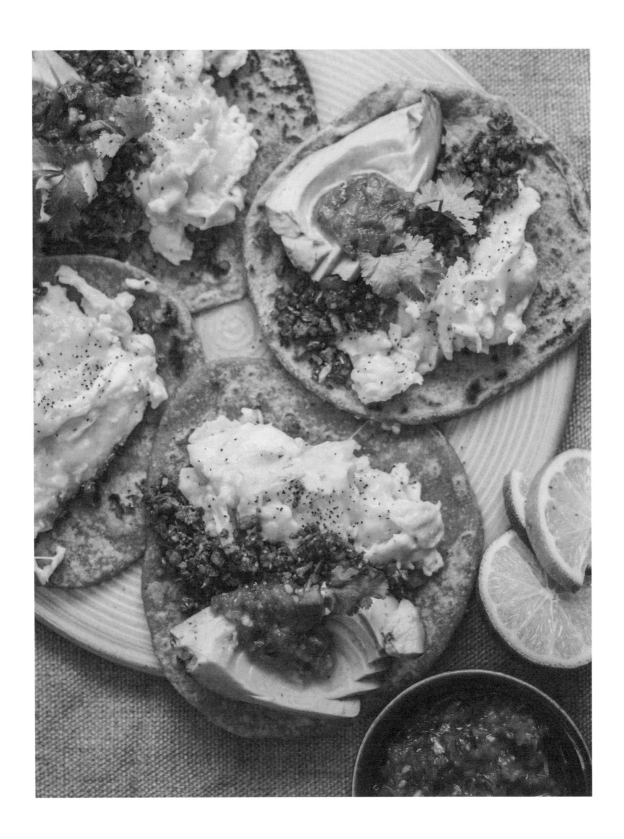

Curried Tofu Scramble

A vegan alternative to scrambled eggs, this tofu scramble can be enjoyed on its own or used in another dish, such as our Breakfast Tacos (p. 46).

SERVES 4

14 ounces firm tofu, drained

1 tablespoon canola oil

1 onion, finely chopped

1 green bell pepper, finely chopped

1 teaspoon curry powder

⅛ teaspoon ground turmeric (optional)

¼ teaspoon kosher salt

Squeeze tofu block in a clean kitchen towel over the sink to remove some of its water. Using your hands, crumble tofu into bite-sized pieces and set aside.

Heat oil in a skillet over medium heat. Add onion and bell pepper. Sauté for about 5 minutes, or until golden brown. Add curry powder and turmeric, if desired. Stir until onion is coated and spices have a chance to bloom, about 30 seconds.

Add crumbled tofu and salt, stirring gently to combine. Cook for 1–2 more minutes, or until tofu is warmed through. Enjoy as you would scrambled eggs—on their own or in a recipe.

Baked Blueberry Oatmeal Bites

Overnight oatmeal meets baked oatmeal in these blueberry-studded muffins. Ideal for breakfast or a snack, these are a convenient, healthy grab-and-go option. Raspberries or finely chopped rhubarb can be used in place of blueberries.

MAKES 12 REGULAR-SIZED MUFFINS

2½ cups rolled oats

¼ cup freshly ground flaxseed

1 teaspoon ground cinnamon

¼ teaspoon table salt

1½ cups milk

¼ cup maple syrup

1 teaspoon pure vanilla extract

1 large egg, beaten

2 tablespoons canola oil

1 teaspoon baking powder

1 cup frozen or fresh blueberries

Mix together oats, flaxseed, cinnamon, and salt in a large bowl. Add the milk, maple syrup, and vanilla, and mix well to combine. Cover and refrigerate overnight or at least 8 hours.

Preheat your oven to 375°F. Lightly oil a regular-sized, 12-cup muffin tin.

Add egg, oil, and baking powder to the soaked oats. You can mix the blueberries into the batter now or wait to use them as a topping just before baking.

Fill prepared muffin tin with oatmeal mixture, about ¼ cup per muffin cup. If you have not already mixed the blueberries into the batter, top each muffin with 1 heaping tablespoon berries.

Bake for 25 minutes, or until muffins are set and tops are just starting to brown. Let muffins cool for 10 minutes before removing from the pan. A table knife might make removal easier.

Once completely cooled, refrigerate in an airtight container for up to 2 days or freeze for up to 3 months. Frozen muffins can be thawed in the microwave for about 30 seconds.

Simple Granola

Adjust ingredients per your taste preferences or according to what you have on hand. Feel free to use any combination of nuts, dried fruits, and seeds. Enjoy this on top of plain yogurt with berries for breakfast or as a between-meal snack.

MAKES 4 CUPS

---

2 cups rolled oats

½ cup chopped pecans

½ cup chopped walnuts

⅓ cup shelled sunflower seeds

2 tablespoons sesame seeds

¼ cup canola or sunflower oil

¼ cup maple syrup or honey

¼ teaspoon table salt

½ cup dried fruit such as raisins, cranberries, cherries, or shredded coconut

Mix oats, nuts, seeds, oil, syrup, and salt together in a medium bowl. Stir until everything is well coated.

Spread the mixture evenly on a baking sheet. (Optional: line baking sheet with eco-friendly parchment for easier cleanup.) Place in a cold oven and turn to 325°F. Start timing and bake for about 30 minutes, or until lightly browned. For even browning, give a stir after halfway through the cooking time.

Remove from oven. Stir in dried fruit. Let cool. Store in an airtight container for up to 1 week or freeze for a much longer shelf life. Simply take out the portion you want when you need it.

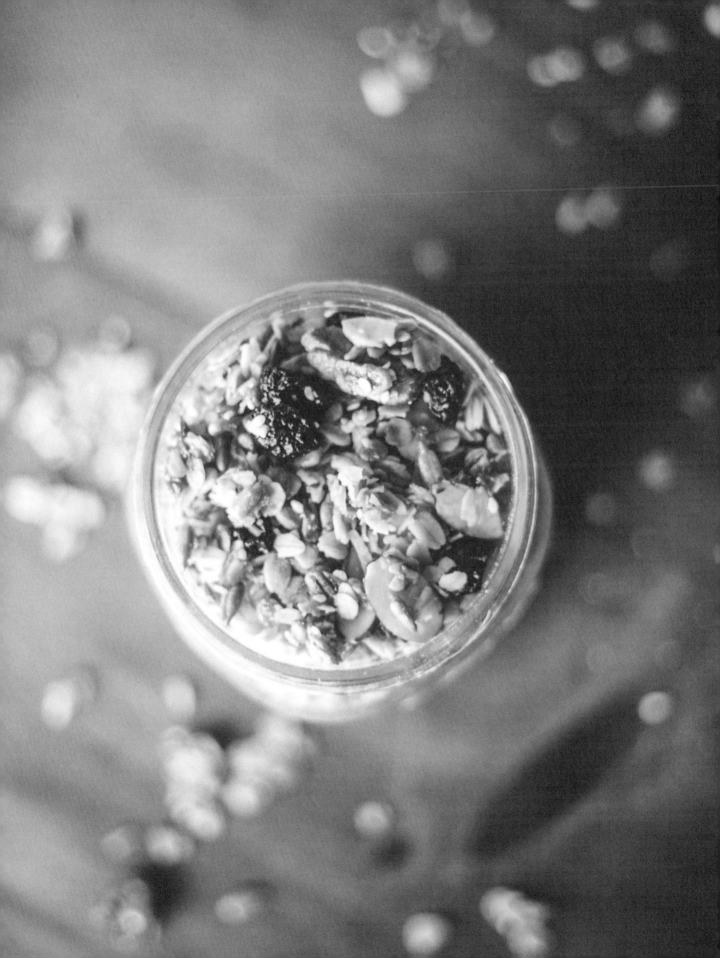

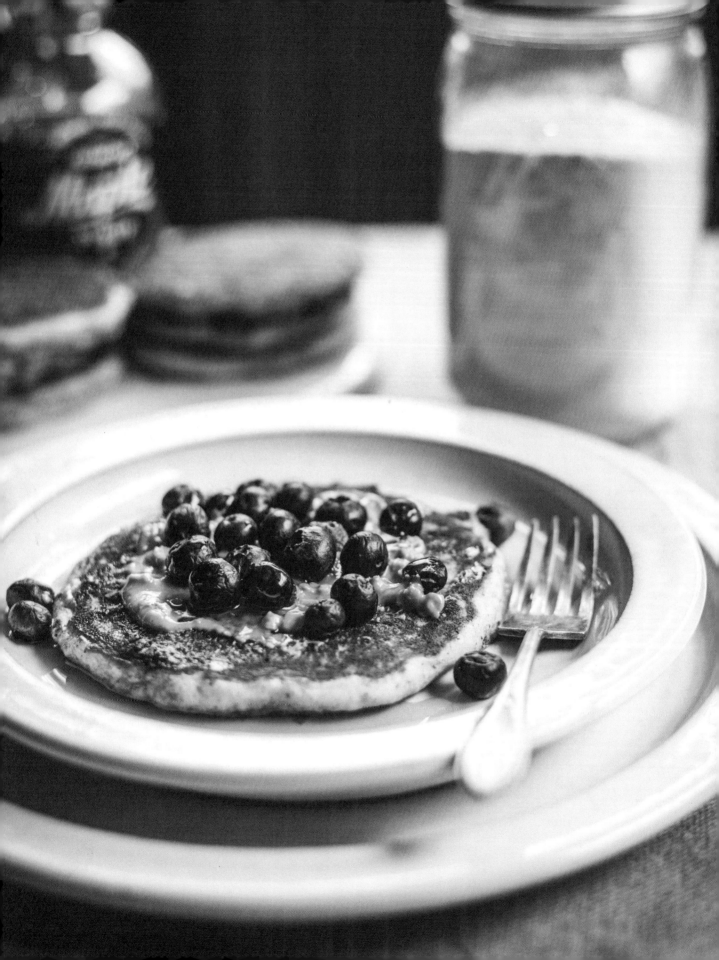

Whole Grain Pancakes or Waffles

Prepare this 100 percent whole grain dry mix ahead of time and store in the freezer. Then, whenever you want pancakes or waffles, just measure your mix and add in the wet ingredients.

Dry Mix

MAKES 4 CUPS

2½ cups (318 grams) white whole wheat flour

1 cup (115 grams) whole grain flour blend; or additional 1 cup (127 grams) white whole wheat

¼ cup freshly ground flaxseed

¼ cup baking powder

1 teaspoon table salt

Precisely measure the flours (technique on p. 310–311). Whisk together ingredients. If you plan to use the mixture soon, store in an airtight container at room temperature; otherwise, store in the refrigerator or freezer for optimal freshness. When you are ready to make pancakes or waffles, proceed to the next page for additional ingredients and directions.

NOTE: There are many whole grain flour blends available, generally incorporating anywhere from six to twelve grains. You can also create your own mix.

(continued next page)

Pancakes or Waffles

MAKES 10 (4-INCH) PANCAKES OR
2 (7-INCH) WAFFLES

1 cup milk, buttermilk, whey, or plain yogurt

1 egg

2 tablespoons canola oil

1 tablespoon maple syrup

1 teaspoon pure vanilla extract (optional)

1 cup (130 grams) dry mix (above)

In a large mixing bowl, whisk together milk, egg, oil, syrup, and vanilla, if desired. Precisely measure out the mix using the same technique as for flour. Whisk in 1 cup of the dry mix until just combined (avoid overmixing; some lumps are okay).

Heat a lightly oiled griddle (for pancakes) or waffle iron (for waffles).

For pancakes: Pour a bit less than ¼ cup batter per pancake onto the preheated skillet. Cook 1–2 minutes per side, or until golden brown. It is time to flip when the edges are becoming set and lots of air bubbles are visible. If you want any add-ins (like blueberries or shredded apples with cinnamon), sprinkle onto each pancake just before the flip.

For waffles: Pour enough batter to cover the bottom of your preheated waffle iron. Cook according to your waffle iron manufacturer's directions.

Serve with your favorite toppings. Fruits and nuts are nutritious choices. Spread with a thin layer of nut butter with banana slices or berries with a sprinkle of finely chopped nuts. Serve with our Berry Sauce (p. 221) or Strawberry-Rhubarb Compote (p. 227).

MAKE IT YOURSELF

Yogurt (p. 280)
Buttermilk (p. 282)

FOOD AS MEDICINE

When I was diagnosed with postpartum depression and anxiety in 2016, I was immediately prescribed an antidepressant. Knowing it would be temporary, and needing something to help me function day to day, I felt okay with taking it. I trusted the psychiatrist who evaluated me and I knew I was not myself. After trying multiple types of medications and having very adverse reactions, I met with the doctor again and she told me that I could try an alternative route: a plant-based, whole-foods diet and regular exercise. I was a vegetarian already, but I was not always eating whole foods, and I was often turning to sugar for comfort. After a few weeks of regular exercise and eating a whole-foods diet, my postpartum depression symptoms were significantly better. I added regular meetings with a therapist and feel strongly that all of those things together really helped me. I support anyone's decision to take medication for mental health and I am thankful to have a solution that works well for me.

Jaymie

Ancient Grains Hot Cereal

For your next bowl of hot cereal, branch out from traditional oatmeal to less familiar, highly nutritious grains that have been around since ancient times. Quinoa, millet, amaranth, and teff—which are commonly referred to as ancient grains—are technically seeds. If you can't find all of them, use more of the ones you do have. Bob's Red Mill is a great source for grains of all kinds.

SERVES 4

¼ **cup quinoa**

¼ **cup millet**

¼ **cup amaranth**

¼ **cup teff**

4 cups water

milk

maple syrup

OPTIONAL TOPPINGS

ground cinnamon

ground nutmeg

sliced banana

berries

raisins

walnuts

pecans

freshly ground flaxseed

Toast the grains: Put the grains in a dry saucepan over medium heat. Cook for several minutes, stirring often, until grains are toasted and teff begins to crackle.

Carefully add water to the hot saucepan, as it may sizzle and splash. Bring to a boil, then reduce heat to a low simmer. Cook, uncovered, for 20 minutes, or until most of the liquid is absorbed and the grains are tender. Stir occasionally during cooking, especially toward the end, to prevent sticking on the bottom of the pan. Mix in a splash of milk, maple syrup, and any of your favorite toppings.

Leftovers will reheat well if served within a few days.

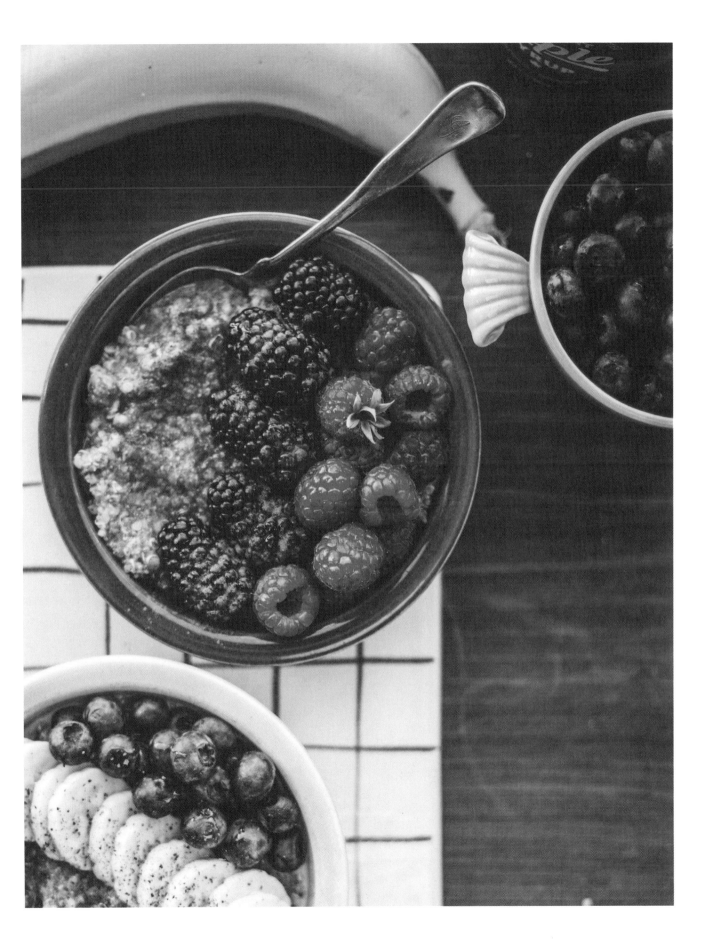

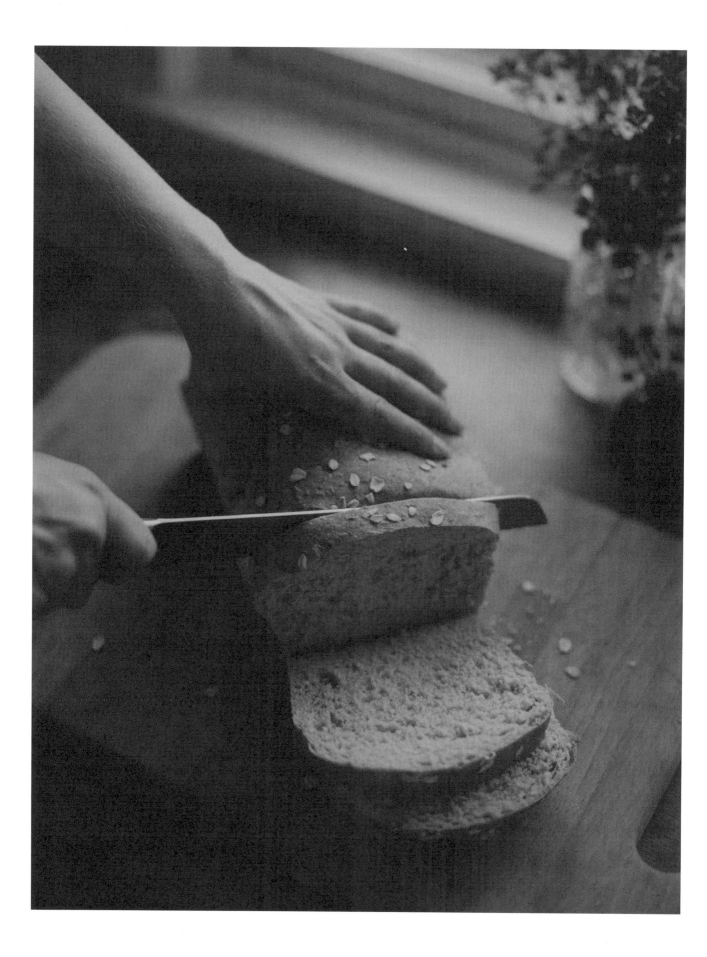

Honey-Oat Breakfast Bread

The process of making bread is wonderful from start to finish. We give instructions for a handmade loaf, but if you happen to have a bread machine, you can put the ingredients into the machine and let it do the rest.

MAKES 1 (2-POUND) LOAF OR 16 (2-OUNCE) SLICES

1½ cups boiling water

1 cup rolled oats

¼ cup honey or maple syrup

2 tablespoons unsalted butter or canola oil

1½ teaspoons table salt

1½ teaspoons instant yeast

1¼ cups (159 grams) whole wheat flour

2¼ cups (277 grams) bread or
all-purpose flour

MAKE IT YOURSELF

Butter (p. 282)

Pour boiling water over oats, honey, butter, and salt in a large bowl. Stir. Allow it to cool until lukewarm. Mix in yeast. Let mixture rest for 5 minutes while you measure the flours (technique on p. 310–311).

Mix flours into the oat-yeast mixture until it starts to come together. This can be done by hand or using a stand mixer with a dough hook attachment. If using a stand mixer, mix for 5 minutes, which will "knead" the dough. If working by hand, turn dough onto a floured surface and knead until it forms a smooth ball. Clean and lightly oil your bowl. Place dough ball in the bowl. Cover with a clean kitchen towel. Let rise for 1½ hours.

Gently push down on the dough to deflate it. Oil a 5 x 10-inch bread loaf pan. Shape dough into a log slightly smaller than the size of your pan. Place the dough log inside the pan. If desired, sprinkle some rolled oats (about 1 tablespoon) on top of the loaf. Cover with the kitchen towel. Let rise for 1 hour.

During the last 10–15 minutes of the second rise, preheat oven to 350°F. Bake for 35–40 minutes until crust is an even golden color. Turn bread out onto a cooling rack. Enjoy some warm slices! Cool completely before storing.

Maple Walnut French Toast

Encrusting French toast with nuts takes breakfast to the next level. This is a great way to start your day, with a nutritious mix of protein, healthy fats, and whole grain carbohydrates. The indulgence comes with butter and syrup, depending how much you add! We recommend using our homemade bread. You can substitute other bread; the amount of egg-milk mixture you need may vary.

MAKES 8 SLICES

2 eggs

½ cup milk

½ teaspoon ground cinnamon

½ teaspoon pure vanilla extract

8 (2-ounce) slices Honey-Oat Breakfast Bread (p. 59) or other bread

1 cup finely chopped walnuts, pecans, or a mix

butter to grease skillet

maple syrup for serving

In a medium bowl, whisk together eggs, milk, cinnamon, and vanilla. Pour into a shallow dish, wide enough to fit a slice of bread.

Preheat griddle or skillet over medium-low heat and grease lightly with butter. Dip each slice of bread in the egg mixture, one at a time, coating both sides. Place as many slices as will comfortably fit on the preheated skillet. Sprinkle nuts evenly over top of each slice of bread, about 2 tablespoons per slice.

Cook about 1 minute per side, or until starting to brown. Flip and press, nut side down, onto skillet for good contact and browning. Serve with maple syrup. Garnish with fresh berries or serve with our Berry Sauce (p. 221) or Strawberry-Rhubarb Compote (p. 227), if desired.

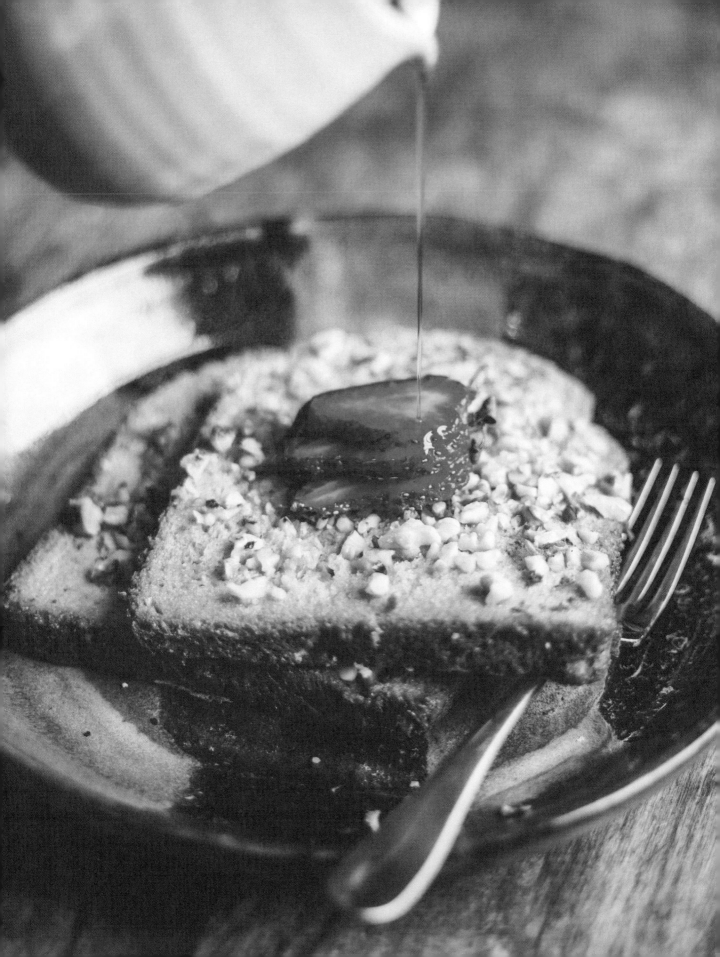

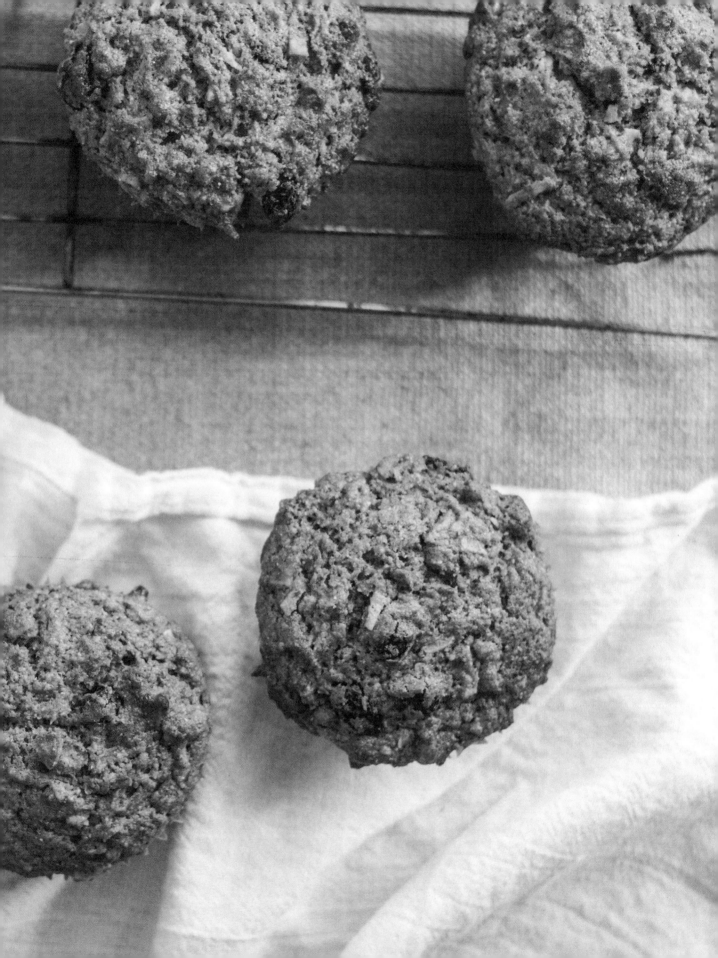

Morning Glory Muffins

A great way to start your day, these portable packages have everything you need to be nourished. Healthy never tasted better than this moist, perfectly spiced, and subtly sweetened muffin.

MAKES 12 MUFFINS

---

2 cups (254 grams) white whole wheat or whole wheat flour

2 teaspoons baking soda

2 teaspoons ground cinnamon

½ teaspoon ground ginger

½ teaspoon table salt

1½ cups grated carrot

1 cup grated apple

½ cup raisins

½ cup finely chopped walnuts

⅓ cup shredded unsweetened coconut

¼ cup freshly ground flaxseed or whole shelled sunflower seeds

3 eggs

¾ cup honey or maple syrup

⅔ cup canola oil

¼ cup orange juice (juice of 1 small orange)

2 teaspoons pure vanilla extract

Preheat oven to 375°F. Lightly oil a 12-cup muffin tin.

Measure the flour (technique on p. 310–311). In a large bowl, mix together flour, baking soda, cinnamon, ginger, and salt. Stir in carrot, apple, raisins, walnuts, coconut, and flaxseed.

In a small bowl, whisk together eggs, honey, oil, orange juice, and vanilla. Add these wet ingredients to the large bowl and mix everything together until evenly distributed.

Fill muffin cups to the top with batter. Bake for about 25 minutes, or until a toothpick inserted in the center of a muffin comes out clean.

Let muffins cool in the tin for 5 minutes before removing. Cool completely before storing in an airtight container (muffins will keep up to several days at room temperature, or several months in the freezer).

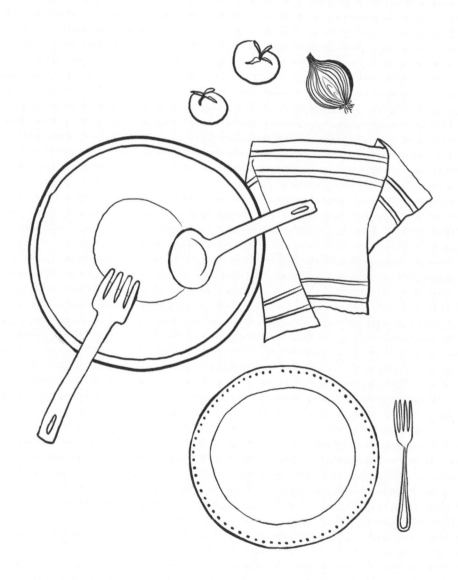

Salads

———

Cobb Salad

This protein-packed salad was named after a restaurant owner, Richard Cobb. Legend has it that Cobb had not eaten until near midnight, so he mixed together leftovers he found in the kitchen. This salad would definitely satisfy a big appetite!

SERVES 2 AS A MAIN DISH OR 4 AS A SIDE

---

4 packed cups chopped romaine lettuce or other salad greens, washed and dried

½ cup Avocado Dressing (p. 261) or Buttermilk Ranch Dressing (p. 265)

4 hard-cooked eggs, sliced; or 1½ cups cooked chickpeas

1 cup chopped tomatoes

1 cup fresh or frozen corn kernels, thawed

2 ounces cheddar cheese, shredded or shaved

1 cup julienned vegetables (such as carrots, red pepper, red onion)

sunflower seeds, to garnish

Place the lettuce in a large bowl and toss with the dressing. Top the salad with eggs or chickpeas, tomatoes, corn, cheese, and your choice of vegetables. Garnish with sunflower seeds.

NOTE: One method that works well for hard-cooked eggs—even for freshly laid eggs that can otherwise be hard to peel—is to steam them for 16 minutes in a steamer basket inside a covered saucepan. Start timing once the steam has built up and is starting to escape from under the lid. When the timer goes off, immediately plunge steamed eggs into an ice bath. Once cool, the eggs are ready to peel and slice.

Zesty Garlic Kale Salad

A salad in which the only vegetable is kale—and it's not even boring! Enjoy as is or use in our Roasted Veggie and Chickpea Bowl (p. 150).

SERVES 4

---

1 (8-ounce) bunch kale

½ cup Lemon Garlic Tahini Dressing (p. 266)

sesame seeds for garnish

Remove and compost kale stems. Wash and dry leaves. Chop or tear into bite-sized pieces.

Add the prepared kale to a large salad bowl. Add about three-quarters of the dressing and gently massage it into the kale leaves with your fingertips. Taste. Add more dressing per your preference.

Toast sesame seeds, if desired (technique on p. 312), and use for garnish.

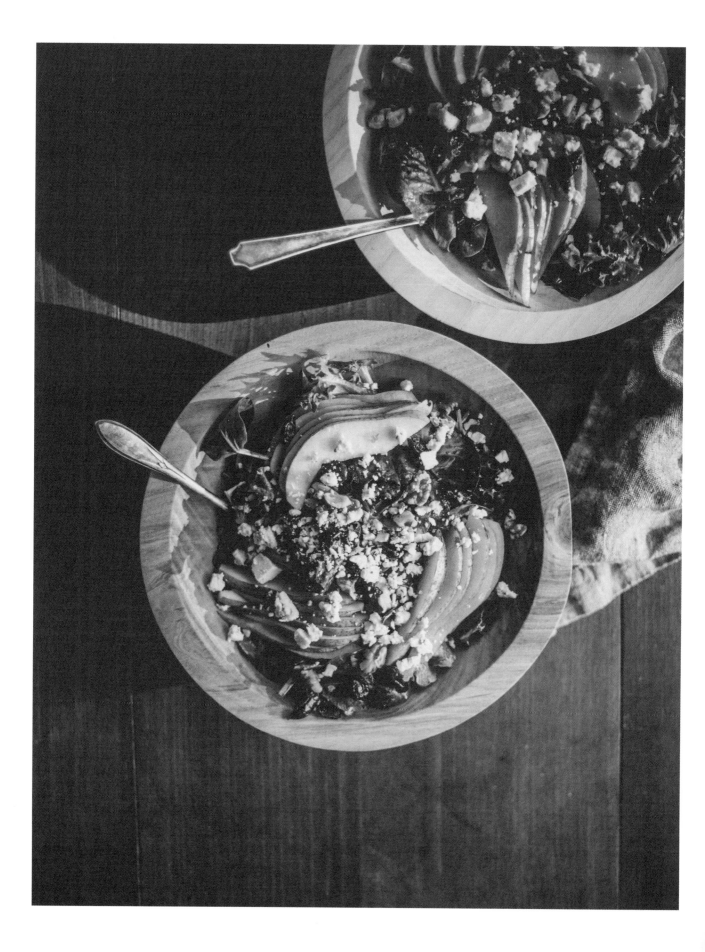

Pear Walnut Salad

The contrast of sweet fruit and strong cheese is complementary in this hearty salad. Tossing your salad greens with the dressing, rather than drizzling it over the top, ensures that every bite has uniformly pleasant flavor.

SERVES 4

8 ounces salad greens, washed and dried

⅔ cup balsamic Vinaigrette (p. 260)

2 pears, cored and sliced

½ cup walnuts or Maple Candied Walnuts (p. 216)

¼ cup dried cranberries

4 ounces Gorgonzola cheese, crumbled

Just before serving, toss greens with about half the vinaigrette until leaves are evenly coated. Top with pear slices, walnuts, dried cranberries, and Gorgonzola cheese. Serve remaining dressing on the side.

Roasted Beet and Goat Cheese Salad or Sandwich

When roasted, earthy beets start to caramelize and develop rich flavor. Pair with creamy goat cheese and some tender greens for a truly special salad, or make it a sandwich with hummus (see variation below).

SERVES 4

SALAD

4 medium red or golden beets

1 tablespoon olive oil

¼ teaspoon kosher salt

⅛ teaspoon freshly ground black pepper

8 ounces salad greens, washed and dried

⅔ cup balsamic Vinaigrette (p. 260)

2-4 ounces goat cheese

SANDWICH

4 whole wheat pitas

All salad ingredients except balsamic Vinaigrette

½ cup Classic Hummus (p. 251)

Wash beets and trim off both tops and bottoms. You can leave the skin on. Cut medium-sized beets vertically into quarters. (Small beets can be halved and large beets cut into 8 slices.) Place beets in a small bowl and toss with olive oil, salt, and pepper. Stir until evenly coated.

Spread the beets on a baking sheet. Place in a cold oven and turn to 450°F. Start timing. Roast in the oven for 35–45 minutes, until a knife inserts easily through the beets. Remove from oven and set aside.

Salad: Just before serving, toss salad greens with about half the vinaigrette until leaves are evenly coated. Top with roasted beets and crumbled goat cheese. Add more vinaigrette as desired.

Sandwich: Using 4 whole wheat pitas, cut pitas in half and spread 2 tablespoons of hummus inside each pita pocket half. Slice the roasted beet wedges so they fit easily inside the pita, using about one beet per pita. Sprinkle in some goat cheese and add some dry salad greens (without vinaigrette).

NOTE: Save beet greens for Beet Green Sauté (p. 182) or a variation on Carrot Top Pesto (p. 248).

Summer Berry and Spinach Salad

A beautiful summer salad with nuts and fresh berries adorning tender dark leafy greens.

SERVES 4

½ cup sliced raw almonds or chopped walnuts (about 2 ounces)

½ cup Poppy Seed Dressing (p. 259) or balsamic Vinaigrette (p. 260)

8 ounces baby spinach or other salad greens, washed and dried

2 cups sliced strawberries

1 cup blueberries

4 ounces goat or feta cheese, crumbled

Toast the nuts (technique on p. 312). Alternatively, make maple candied walnuts (p. 216).

In a large mixing bowl, toss greens with the dressing or vinaigrette until leaves are evenly coated. Top each salad with berries, nuts, and goat cheese.

Eat Your "Weeds" Salad

We are surrounded by an edible landscape with many plants that we label as "weeds" being nutrient rich and safe for human consumption. Learning more about your native flora and how to use what grows naturally is important to resiliency and sourcing a sustainable food supply. Rather than expend great effort trying to rid your lawn or garden of "weeds," embrace this free perennial food source that requires no effort on your part. The prospect of eating your "weeds" is a great reason to practice organic lawn and garden care. Each "weed" will have its own unique flavor profile—for example, sorrels offer a sour lemony flavor. Have fun exploring your backyard and what it has to offer.

YIELD VARIES

Local edible "weeds," which may include:

young dandelion leaves and flowers

red clover leaves and flowers

violet leaves and flowers

purslane, remove thick stem

trefoil (wood sorrel), upper half

sheep sorrel leaves

chickweed, upper leaf portion

lambsquarter leaves

OPTIONAL ADD-INS

any other salad greens and vegetables

toasted nuts (technique on p. 312)

boiled eggs

croutons

DRESSING

3 parts oil, such as extra-virgin olive oil

1 part acid, such as freshly squeezed lemon juice or red wine vinegar

kosher salt and freshly ground black pepper

minced garlic (optional)

Harvest your "weeds" as close to serving time as you can. Only pick what you plan to use that day.

Wash well in cold water and dry in a salad spinner, or simply allow to drain. Store in refrigerator until ready to use, although it is ideal to prepare and eat them immediately.

Prepare any optional ingredients you wish to add.

Prepare dressing using suggested 3:1 ratio of oil to acid, which is a classic formula for simple vinaigrettes. Season with salt and pepper to taste. Add garlic, if desired. Whisk all dressing ingredients in a small bowl or shake them together in a jar with a tight-fitting lid.

Mix "weeds" with any optional add-ins. Toss salad with enough dressing to coat the leaves. Serve additional dressing on the side.

MAKE IT YOURSELF

Croutons (p. 291)

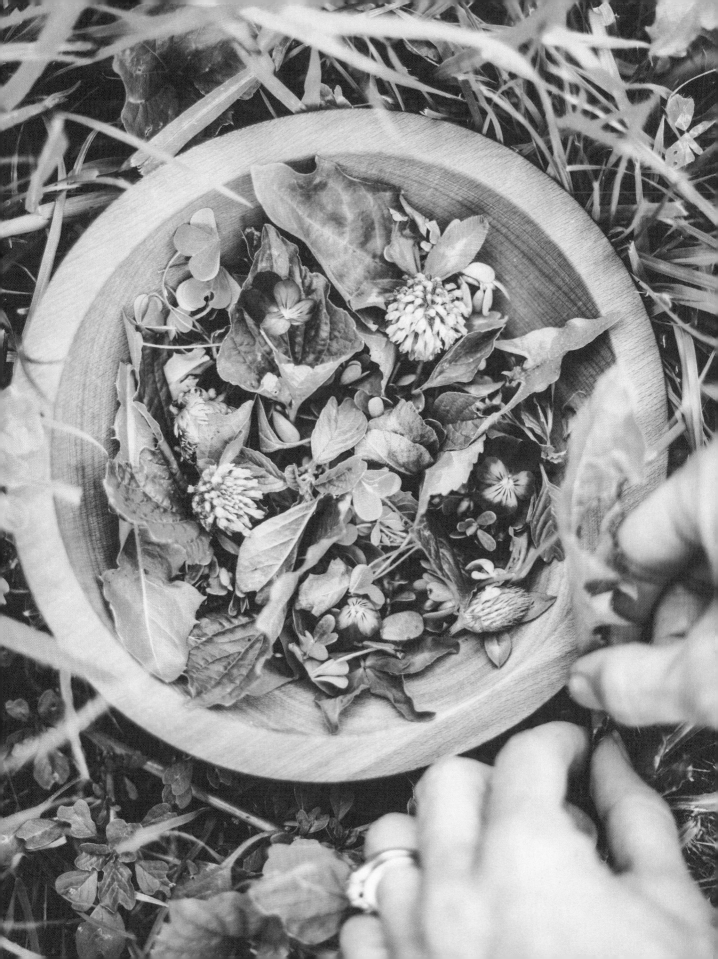

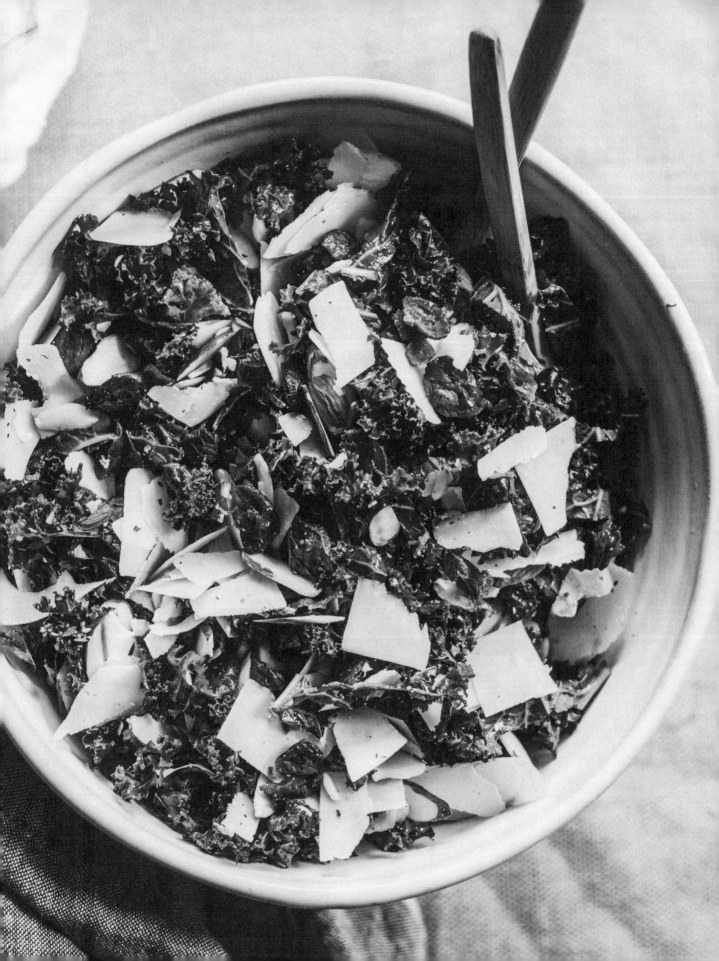

Lemony Kale Salad

Raw kale cut thinly into little ribbons makes this hearty green more tender on the tongue. **Chiffonade** *is the term for this knife technique for cutting greens and herbs. Massaging the simple lemon-and-oil dressing into the greens using your hands also tenderizes the kale.*

SERVES 6

1 (8-ounce) bunch kale

juice of ½ lemon

2 tablespoons extra-virgin olive oil

⅛ teaspoon kosher salt

⅛ teaspoon freshly ground black pepper

½ cup slivered (or sliced) almonds

½ cup shredded or shaved (not grated) Parmesan cheese

⅓ cup dried cranberries

Remove and compost kale stems. Wash and dry leaves.

Chiffonade the kale by making a small stack of the leaves and rolling them up. Thinly slice the leaves crosswise into little ribbons of kale. Place kale ribbons in a large bowl.

Whisk together lemon juice, oil, salt, and pepper.

Add dressing to kale. Mix well to coat all leaves and massage the dressing into the kale.

Top the salad with almonds, Parmesan cheese, and dried cranberries.

Cruciferous Cranberry Crunch Salad

Cruciferous vegetables—such as broccoli, cauliflower, cabbage, kale, arugula, brussels sprouts, and radishes—get their name from the Latin **cruciferae***, meaning "cross bearing," because their flowers have four petals that resemble a cross. You can make this salad using kale or brussels sprouts.*

SERVES 6

1 (8-ounce) bunch kale; or 15 brussels sprouts

1½ cups finely chopped or shredded red cabbage

1½ cups julienned or shredded carrots (about 2 carrots)

1 stem broccoli (no florets), julienned or shredded (optional)

⅔ cup red wine Vinaigrette (p. 260) or ½ cup Poppy Seed Dressing (p. 259)

½ cup dried cranberries

½ cup chopped walnuts or whole shelled sunflower seeds

½ cup crumbled feta cheese (optional)

If using kale, remove and compost stems, wash and dry leaves, then chop finely. If using raw brussels sprouts, thinly shave them. A mandoline works well for this task of making very thin slices.

Combine kale or brussels sprouts, cabbage, carrots, and optional broccoli in a large salad bowl. Toss with vinaigrette. Plate and top with dried cranberries, walnuts, and optional feta cheese.

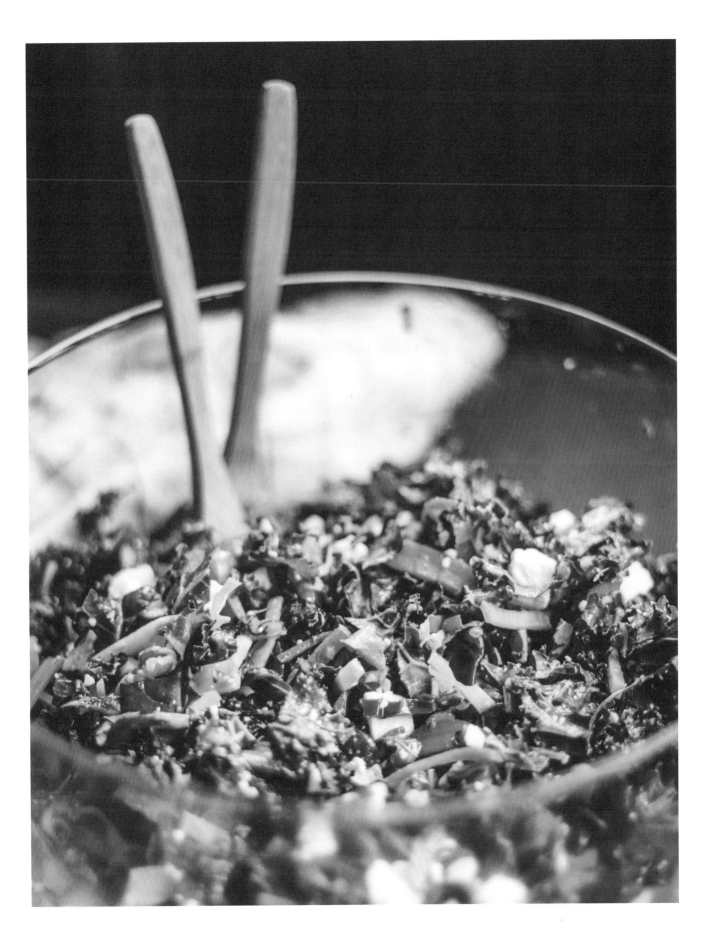

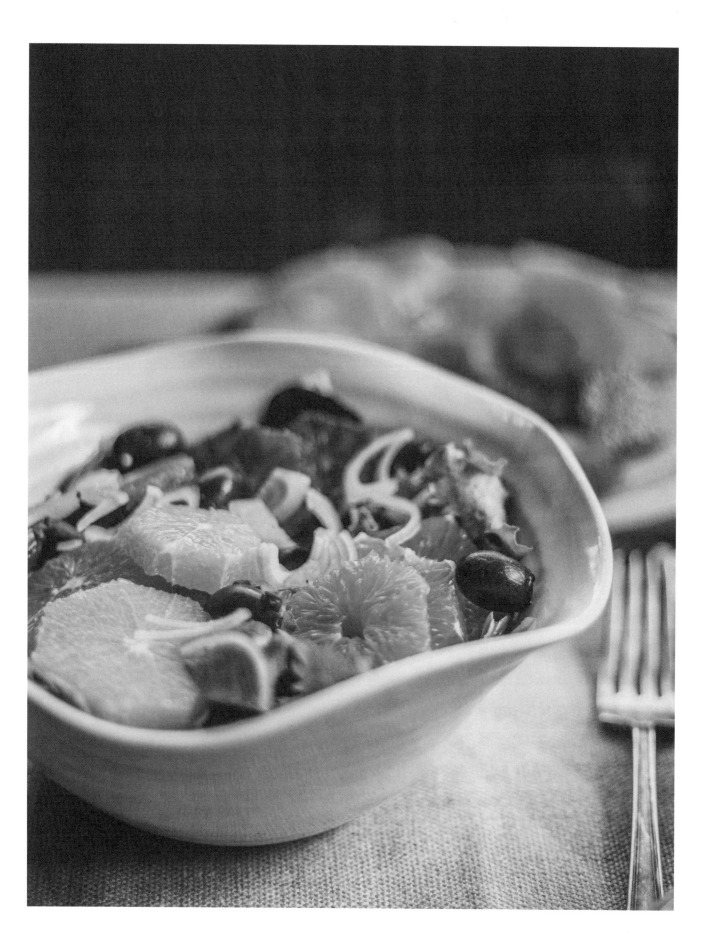

Citrus Salad

Citrus brings us a touch of sunshine, especially in winter months. Cara Cara, navel, and blood oranges make a pretty combination of pink, orange, and red in this salad. You can also substitute white, red, and pink grapefruit if desired.

SERVES 4

2 tablespoons red wine vinegar or lemon juice

2 teaspoons extra-virgin olive oil

2 teaspoons minced shallot

¼ teaspoon salt

¼ teaspoon freshly ground black pepper

⅛ teaspoon cayenne or smoked paprika (optional)

5 ounces salad greens, washed and dried

4 cups orange slices (about 2 pounds)

½ cup pitted kalamata olives

thinly sliced red onion, shallot, or fennel (optional)

Whisk together a dressing of vinegar, oil, 2 teaspoons shallot, salt, and pepper. If you like spicy flavors, add cayenne or smoked paprika for some kick.

Just before serving, mix dressing with salad greens. Top with oranges and olives. If desired, add onion, shallot, or fennel.

Greek Cucumber Chopped Salad

This refreshing side salad features fresh crisp cucumbers. A juicy ripe tomato will naturally add liquid to the simple dressing of olive oil, vinegar, and herbs. Serve alongside Classic Hummus (p. 251) and whole grain pita to make it a meal.

SERVES 4

2 cups chopped cucumber

1 tomato, chopped

½ cup crumbled feta cheese

¼ cup pitted and chopped kalamata olives

¼ cup finely chopped red onion or shallot

2 tablespoons extra-virgin olive oil

1 tablespoon red wine vinegar

1 tablespoon minced fresh dill weed; or
1 teaspoon dried

2 teaspoons chopped fresh oregano; or
½ teaspoon dried

⅛ teaspoon freshly ground black pepper
(optional)

Combine all ingredients in a large bowl. Toss gently until well coated.

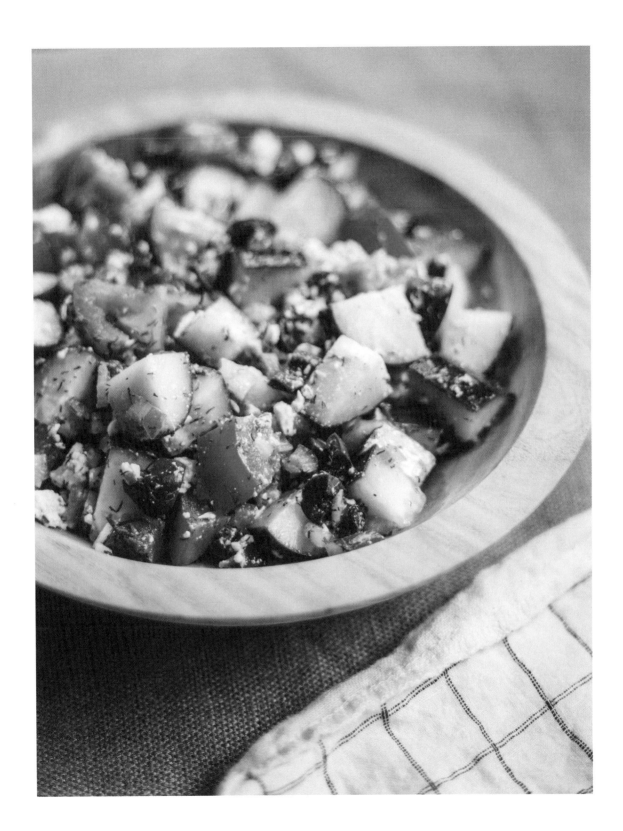

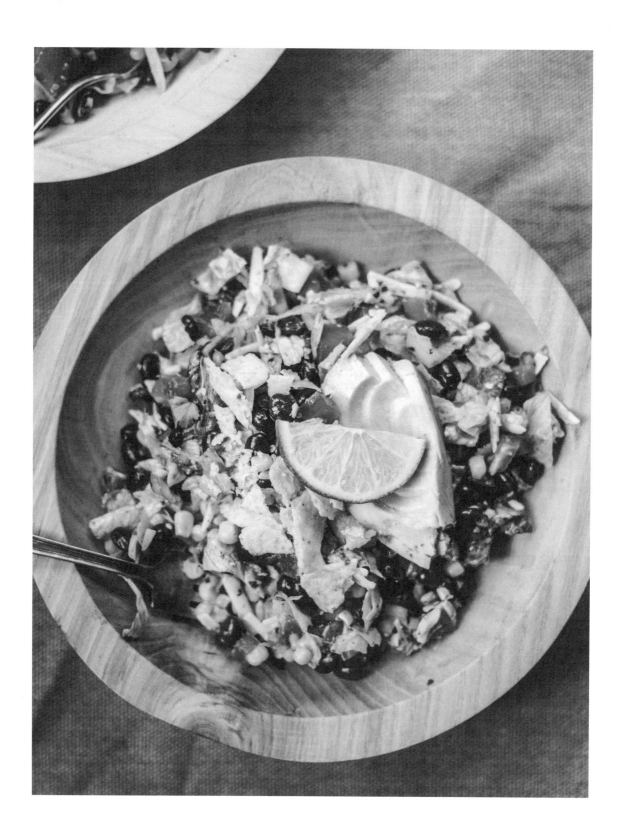

Southwest Chopped Salad

A simple salad that requires minimal effort and is most satisfying on a summer's day. The Cilantro Lime Dressing is preferred for this recipe; use parsley as a substitute for anyone with a cilantro aversion.

SERVES 4

1½ cups cooked black beans

2 cups chopped romaine lettuce or other salad greens, washed and dried

1 cup corn kernels

½ cup finely chopped red bell pepper

1 avocado, chopped

1 tomato, chopped

2 tablespoons finely chopped green onions or red onion

2 ounces cheddar cheese, shredded

¾ cup Cilantro Lime Dressing (p. 262) or Avocado Dressing (p. 261)

1 cup crushed tortilla chips (optional)

Combine beans, romaine, corn, bell pepper, avocado, tomato, green onions, and cheddar cheese in a large bowl. Add a ½ cup of the dressing and toss the salad gently until romaine leaves are evenly coated with dressing. Serve remaining dressing on the side and add more as desired.

Top with crushed tortilla chips for extra crunch, if desired.

Edamame Caprese Salad

Caprese (tomato, mozzarella, basil) is a refreshing salad. This version gets a nutritional boost from the addition of high-fiber, protein-rich edamame, which are young, green soybeans. Eat as a simple snack or side salad. Make it a meal by mixing into cooked pasta or whole grains.

SERVES 6

---

2 cups shelled fresh or frozen edamame (about 10 ounces)

8 ounces fresh mozzarella cheese, cut into bite-sized pieces

2 large tomatoes, chopped

½ cup Classic Basil Pesto (p. 247)

kosher salt and freshly ground pepper

pine nuts for garnish

In a medium saucepot, bring ½ cup water to a boil. Add edamame, cover, and return to a boil over medium-high heat. Boil for about 6 minutes. Drain and rinse under cold water.

Mix together edamame, mozzarella cheese, tomatoes, and pesto. Taste. If desired, top with a little salt and pepper.

Toast the nuts (technique on p. 312). Use to garnish salad.

Seven Cs Couscous Salad

Seven ingredients in this salad start with the letter C. Make this recipe for others and invite them to guess the seven. This practice cultivates mindful eating: becoming more aware of our food by slowing down and engaging all our senses. Paying close attention to flavors and textures helps us appreciate our food.

SERVES 6

---

1 (14-ounce) can unsweetened coconut milk

1 teaspoon curry powder

¼ teaspoon kosher salt

1 cup whole wheat couscous

1 cup grated carrot

½ cup chopped cashews

½ cup currants or dried cranberries

¼ cup chopped fresh cilantro

Combine coconut milk, curry powder, and salt in a medium saucepan. Bring to a boil. Stir in couscous, cover, and remove from heat. Let sit for 5 minutes. Remove cover and fluff couscous with a fork. Stir in carrot, cashews, currants, and cilantro. Serve warm or at room temperature.

Balsamic Three Bean Salad

Three bean salad is a speedy summer side dish that can be as simple as beans and dressing. Try some add-ins for extra color, freshness, flavor, and nutrition. This salad is an easy way to up your intake of legumes, which count as both vegetable and protein in our diets.

SERVES 6

1½ cups cooked kidney beans

1½ cups cooked black beans

1½ cups cooked chickpeas

1 cup fresh or frozen corn or green beans

1 clove garlic, minced

⅔ cup balsamic Vinaigrette (p. 260)

OPTIONAL ADD-INS

¼ cup finely chopped red onion

¼ cup chopped red bell pepper

1 avocado, chopped

1 tomato, chopped

¼ cup minced fresh herbs such as basil or cilantro

lettuce, washed and dried

In a large bowl, combine kidney beans, black beans, chickpeas, corn, garlic, and vinaigrette. Stir until well combined. Cover and refrigerate for at least 4 hours. Flavor will continue to infuse the longer it sits.

Before serving, mix in any or all of the optional add-ins, if desired. Serve as a side dish, or scoop onto lettuce for a salad.

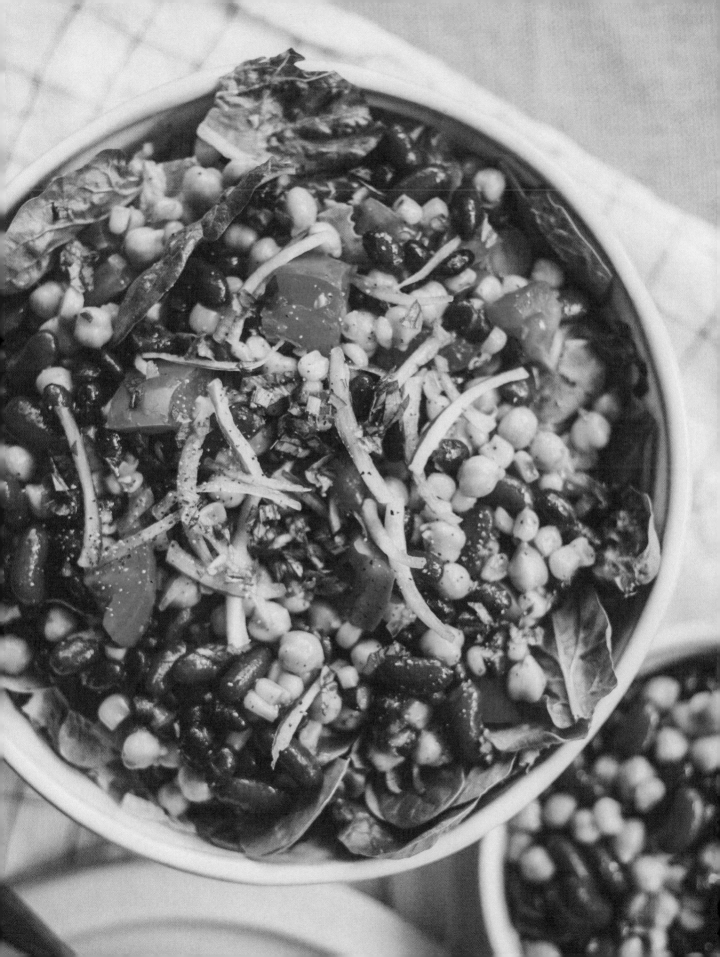

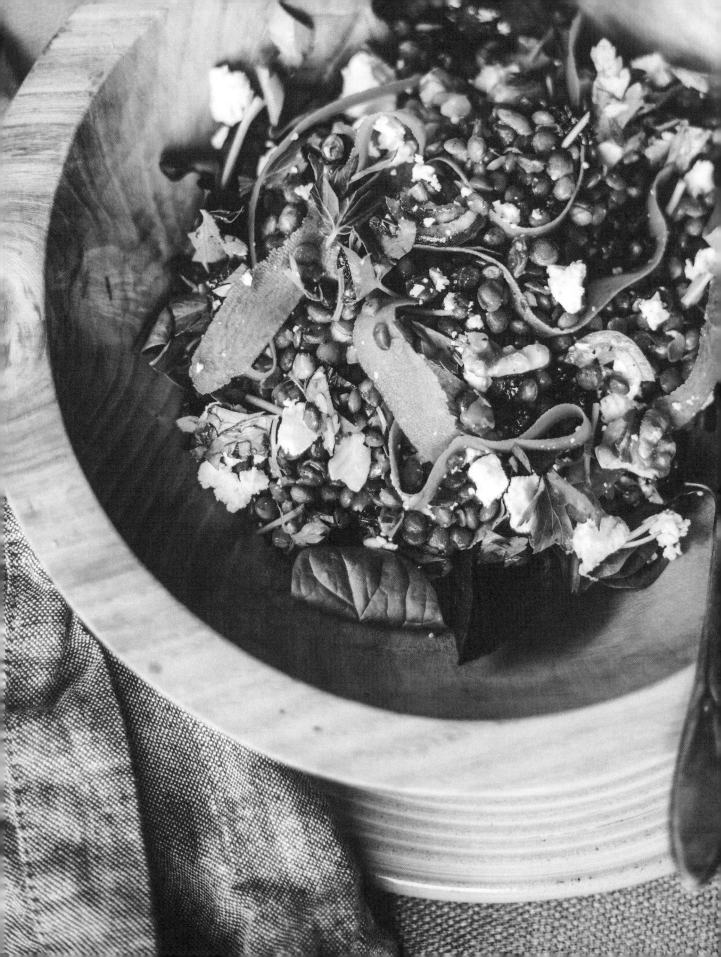

Moroccan Spiced Lentil Salad

Of the different types of lentils, French lentils hold their texture best for cold salads such as this one. The many spices and seasonings make the ingredient list appear long, but all that is required is to simply measure and mix into a dressing.

SERVES 6

SALAD

1 cup green French lentils, sorted and rinsed

4 cups water

⅓ cup dried currants

2 heaping tablespoons capers, drained

½ red onion, finely chopped

5 ounces baby spinach or mesclun greens, washed and dried

DRESSING

2 tablespoons olive oil

2 tablespoons apple cider vinegar

1½ teaspoons maple syrup

1½ teaspoons whole grain, Dijon, or spicy brown mustard

½ teaspoon kosher salt

½ teaspoon ground cumin

¼ teaspoon ground turmeric

¼ teaspoon ground coriander

⅛ teaspoon ground nutmeg

⅛ teaspoon ground cardamom

⅛ teaspoon cayenne

⅛ teaspoon ground cloves

⅛ teaspoon ground cinnamon

⅛ teaspoon freshly ground black pepper

OPTIONAL TOPPINGS

chopped walnuts

crumbled feta or goat cheese

minced fresh cilantro or parsley

chopped cucumber

shredded carrots (or shaved into ribbons)

chopped celery

quartered cherry tomatoes

chopped bell peppers

Place lentils and water in a medium saucepan. Bring to a boil over high heat, then reduce heat to a simmer. Cover and cook until lentils are al dente (cooked through but still firm), about 25 minutes.

Drain lentils in a colander and run them under cold water or put them in a bath of ice water to stop further cooking. You don't want mushy, overcooked lentils in salads.

Whisk all dressing ingredients in a small bowl or shake them together in a jar with a tight-fitting lid.

Combine cooled, drained lentils, dried currants, capers, onion, and dressing together in a large bowl. Serve over salad greens topped with any optional add-ins, if desired.

Wheat Berry, Apple, and Walnut Salad

The chewy wheat berries, crisp apples, and crunchy nuts combine to create a salad full of texture and satisfaction. Wheat berries are the mother grain: wheat in its whole form before it is ground into flour. Substitute any whole form of grains, such as oat groats, rye berries, or spelt berry, or a semi-pearled barley or farro. Adjust cooking time for selected grain (see chart on p. 309).

SERVES 4

_____

SALAD

1 cup winter wheat berries or other whole grain, sorted and rinsed

3 cups water

½ teaspoon kosher salt

1 large apple, cored and diced

½ cup chopped walnuts or pecans, toasted if desired

½ cup dried cranberries or raisins

½ cup minced fresh parsley (optional)

DRESSING

¼ cup extra-virgin olive oil

3 tablespoons apple cider vinegar, freshly squeezed lemon juice, or a combination

½ teaspoon dried thyme; or ¼ teaspoon ground cinnamon plus ¼ teaspoon ground nutmeg

½ teaspoon kosher salt

Put wheat berries, water, and salt in a medium saucepan. Bring to a boil. Reduce heat, cover, and simmer for 1 hour, or until tender. (Alternatively, pressure-cook the wheat berries for 30 minutes followed by a 10-minute natural release.) Drain off any excess water. Set aside to cool.

Combine the cooked wheat berries, apple, nuts, and dried cranberries in a large bowl.

You can go two ways with this dressing. Choose thyme (savory) or cinnamon and nutmeg (sweet). Whisk all dressing ingredients in a small bowl or shake them together in a jar with a tight-fitting lid.

Stir dressing into the salad. Mix in optional parsley, if desired in the savory dressing. Flavors will be best if allowed to stand for 30 minutes before serving.

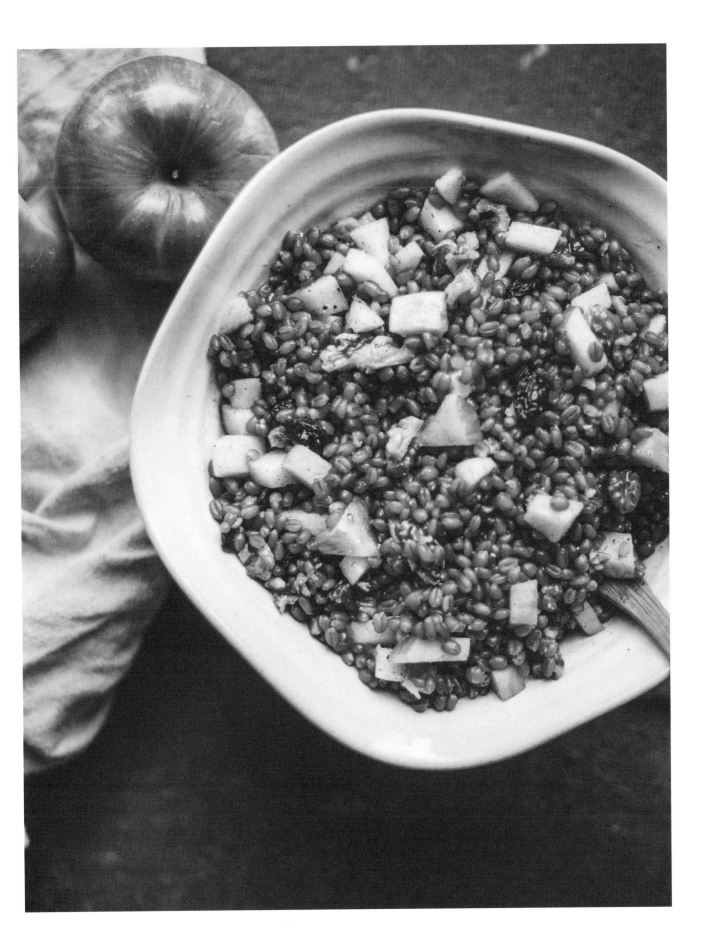

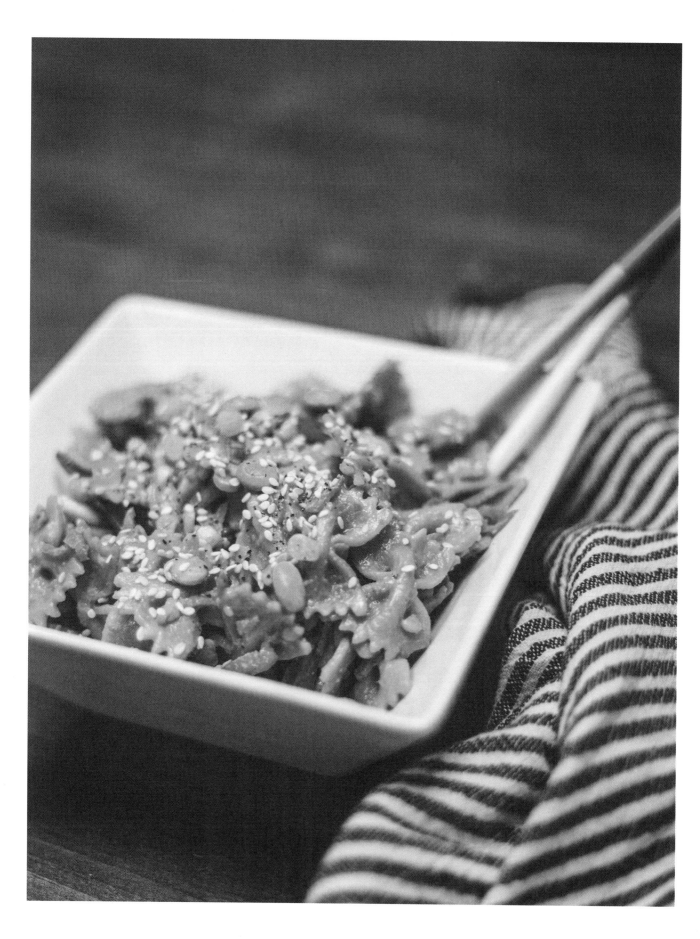

Bow "Thai" Salad

You just can't go wrong with peanut sauce. Feel free to add other veggies you might have on hand.

SERVES 4

8 ounces farfalle (also known as bow-tie or butterfly) pasta or soba (buckwheat) noodles

1 cup frozen or fresh shelled edamame

2 teaspoons toasted sesame oil

1 teaspoon sesame seeds plus additional for garnish

½ cup Peanut Sauce (p. 252)

1 cup shredded carrot

1 cup julienned red bell pepper

¼ cup finely chopped green onions plus additional for garnish

Cook pasta. Set timer for 6 minutes before the pasta should finish cooking. When 6 minutes cooking time remains, add edamame to the boiling water. Drain and rinse pasta and edamame in a colander, using cold water to stop the cooking. Toss with sesame oil and sesame seeds.

Add peanut sauce to pasta and stir until coated. Stir in carrot, bell pepper, and green onions. Garnish with additional sesame seeds and chopped green onions if desired. Can be served chilled or warm.

Timeless Tabbouleh

Authentic Middle Eastern tabbouleh (or tabouli) is made with more herbs and less bulgur than this version. The bulgur needs time to soak in the dressing, but wait to mix in the herbs and vegetables until just before serving time; this will prevent your tabbouleh from getting soggy. Wondering which parsley to use? Flat leaf has more robust taste, and curly is often used for garnishes. Either works here.

SERVES 6

---

1 cup water

¾ teaspoon kosher salt

1 cup bulgur

juice of 1 lemon

¼ cup extra-virgin olive oil

2 cloves garlic, minced

⅛ teaspoon freshly ground black pepper, or to taste

2 tomatoes, finely diced

1 packed cup finely chopped fresh parsley

½ cucumber, finely diced

½ cup grated carrot

½ cup finely chopped green onions

½ cup crumbled feta cheese

¼ cup pitted and chopped kalamata olives

romaine lettuce leaves, separated, washed, and dried (optional)

Bring water and salt to a boil in a medium saucepan. Stir in bulgur. Remove from heat and cover. Let sit for 20 minutes, until slightly softened.

In a small bowl, whisk together lemon juice, olive oil, garlic, and pepper. Add to the bulgur and stir until well combined. Cover and refrigerate 2–3 hours, allowing the bulgur to marinate and continue to absorb liquid.

Just before serving, use a fork to mix in the tomatoes, parsley, cucumber, carrot, green onions, feta cheese, and olives.

Serving suggestion: Serving tabbouleh with lettuce leaves is customary. Add a scoop to the center of a romaine leaf for a traditional and attractive presentation.

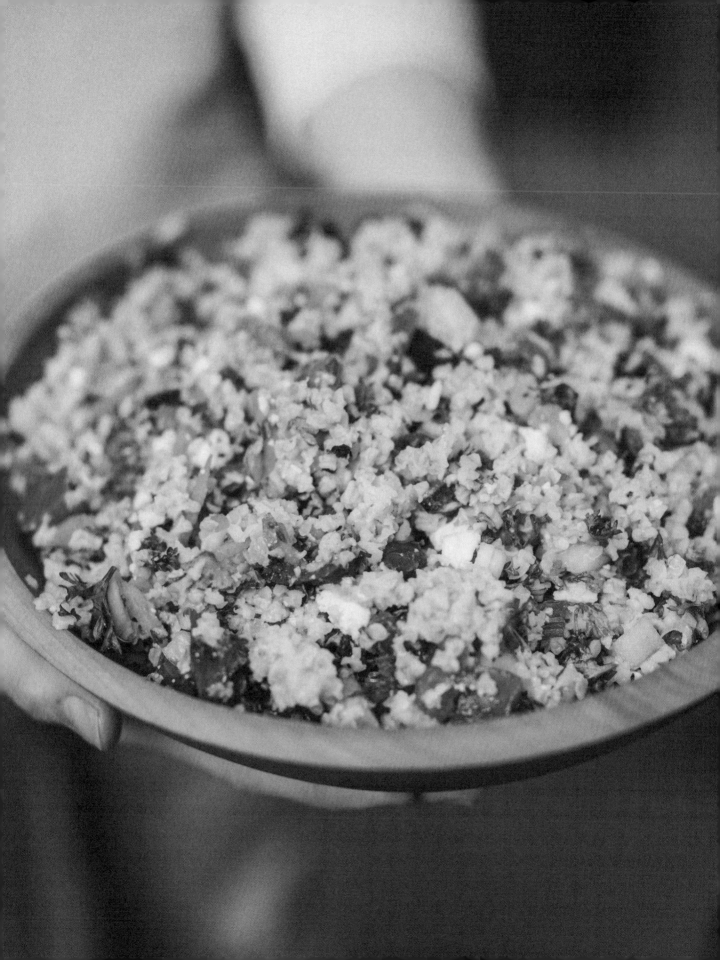

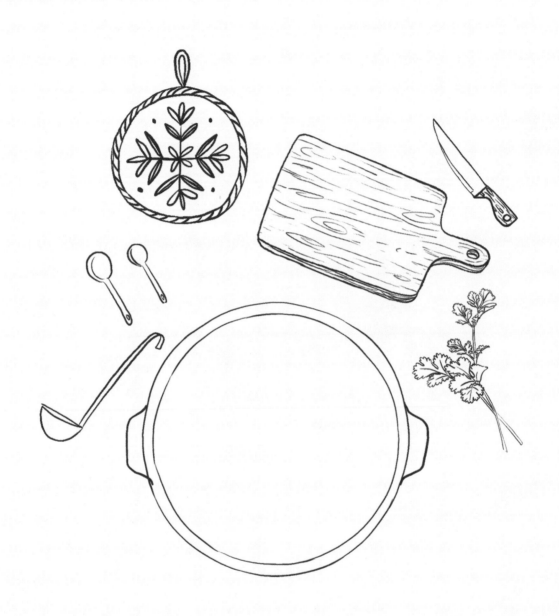

Soups
and Stews

Sweet Potato Chili

Chili powder, cumin, cayenne, cocoa, and cinnamon create a complex flavor blend that warms the mouth with every spoonful. Like most chili recipes, this tastes even better the next day after flavors have a chance to fuse.

SERVES 6

2 tablespoons olive oil

1 onion, chopped

1 red bell pepper, chopped

4 cloves garlic, minced

2 medium sweet potatoes, diced (4–5 cups)

3 cups cooked black or pinto beans or a combination (reserve cooking liquid/aquafaba)

1 cup liquid (reserved aquafaba, broth, or water)

1 (28-ounce) can diced tomatoes; or 4 cups diced fresh

1 tablespoon chili powder

2 teaspoons unsweetened cocoa powder

1½ teaspoons ground cumin

½ teaspoon kosher salt, or to taste

½ teaspoon cayenne, or to taste

¼ teaspoon ground cinnamon

In a large Dutch oven or soup pot, heat oil over medium heat. Add onion and cook for 3 minutes, stirring occasionally. Add bell pepper and cook for another 2–3 minutes. Stir in garlic until fragrant, about 30 seconds. Add all remaining ingredients. Stir to combine.

Bring to a boil, reduce heat, cover, and simmer gently over low heat for 45 minutes, or until sweet potatoes are fork tender. Stir occasionally during cooking. If time allows, let chili sit prior to serving for best flavor.

Slow cooker or multicooker variation: Sauté the onions, pepper, and garlic as above or using the multicooker's sauté function. Add all ingredients to slow cooker or multicooker. Use slow-cook function to cook on low for 6 hours or on high for 3 hours.

MAKE IT YOURSELF

Canned Diced Tomatoes (p. 274)

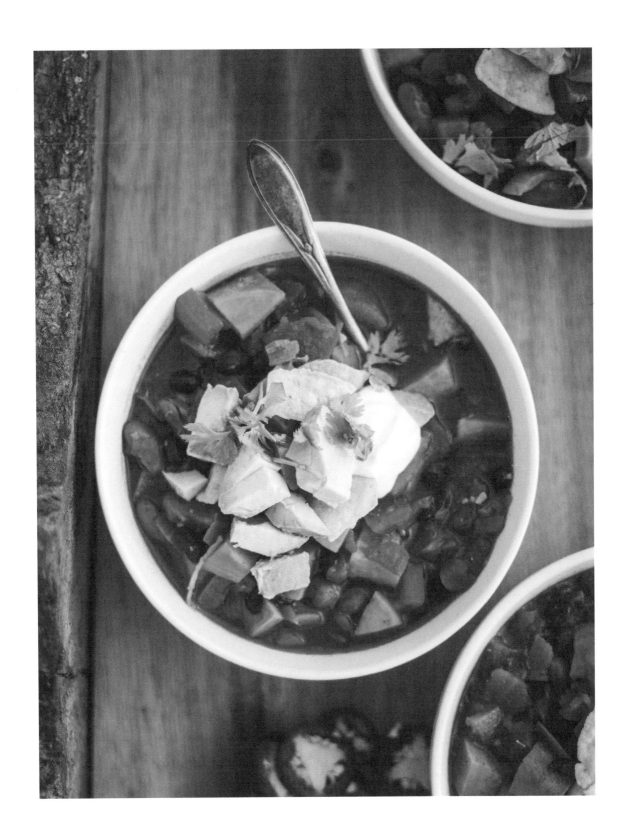

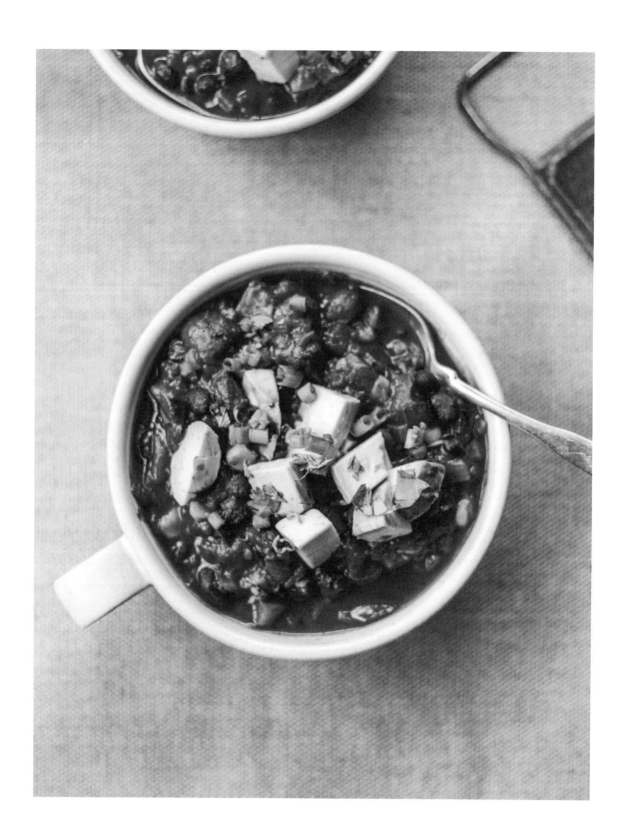

Chipotle Pumpkin Chili

Autumn's favorite vegetable offers a perfect way to herald in the cold fall nights. This is seasoned for a medium level of heat, which can be easily adjusted up or down depending on your taste preferences. Just increase or decrease the amount of chipotle peppers and adobo sauce.

SERVES 6

2 tablespoons olive oil

2 onions, chopped

1 green bell pepper, chopped

4 cloves garlic, minced

1 chipotle pepper in adobo sauce, chopped

2 tablespoons adobo sauce (from the chipotle peppers)

4½ cups cooked black beans

1 (28-ounce) can diced tomatoes (fire roasted are nice); or 4 cups diced fresh

1½ cups plain pumpkin puree

1 cup fresh or frozen corn

1 tablespoon chili powder

1½ teaspoons ground cumin

1 teaspoon kosher salt, or to taste

GARNISHES

sliced avocado

chopped green onions

chopped fresh cilantro

shredded cheddar cheese

In a large Dutch oven or soup pot, heat oil over medium heat. Add onion and cook for 3 minutes over medium heat, stirring occasionally. Add bell pepper and cook for another 2–3 minutes. Stir in garlic until fragrant, 30–60 seconds more. Add all remaining ingredients. Stir to combine. Bring to a boil, reduce heat, cover pot, and simmer gently over low heat for 30 minutes. Stir occasionally during cooking.

If time allows, let chili sit prior to serving for best flavor. Garnish with avocado, green onions, cilantro, and cheddar cheese as desired.

Slow cooker or multicooker variation: Sauté the onions, pepper, and garlic as above or using the multicooker's sauté function. Add all ingredients to slow cooker or multicooker. Cook on low for 6 hours or on high for 3 hours.

MAKE IT YOURSELF

Canned Diced Tomatoes (p. 274)

French Lentil Soup with Kale and Mushrooms

Complex flavors—savory mushrooms, crisp vermouth, slightly sweet shallots, and creamy coconut milk—make this lentil soup unique. Enjoy with some crusty bread on the side.

SERVES 6

3 cups water

1 cup French lentils, sorted and rinsed

kosher salt

1 tablespoon olive oil

1 medium shallot, minced (about ⅓ cup)

1 pound cremini (baby bella) mushrooms, cleaned, trimmed, and sliced

½ teaspoon freshly ground black pepper

2 cloves garlic, minced

1½ teaspoons fresh thyme; or ½ teaspoon dried

2 tablespoons vermouth or dry white wine

2 teaspoons reduced sodium soy sauce or tamari

2 cups liquid (reserved from cooking lentils or vegetable broth)

1½ packed cups thinly sliced kale, stems removed and composted

⅓ cup unsweetened coconut milk (optional)

In a medium saucepan, add water, lentils, and a pinch of salt. Bring to a boil. Reduce heat and simmer, partly covered, for 20–30 minutes (depending on whether you prefer your lentils al dente or soft). Drain lentils, reserving the cooking water, and set both aside.

In a medium soup pot, heat oil over medium heat. Add shallots and cook until softened, about 4 minutes. Add sliced mushrooms and sprinkle with 1 teaspoon salt (or to taste) and pepper. Stir. Cook until the mushrooms begin to glisten, about 3 minutes.

Add garlic and thyme to the pot and stir. Once garlic is fragrant, after about 30 seconds, add vermouth and soy sauce and stir for about another 30 seconds. Stir drained lentils, liquid, kale, and optional coconut milk into the pot.

Bring the soup to a boil. Remove from heat, taste, and adjust seasonings as desired.

MAKE IT YOURSELF

Vegetable Broth (p. 293)

Moroccan Chickpea Stew

A Mediterranean dish inspired by flavors of North Africa, this simple stew can be made on the stovetop or in a multicooker.

SERVES 6

2 tablespoons olive oil

1 onion, chopped

5 cloves garlic, minced

1 teaspoon ground cinnamon

1 teaspoon ground cumin

1 teaspoon paprika

½ teaspoon kosher salt

½ teaspoon freshly ground black pepper

¼ teaspoon ground turmeric

¼ teaspoon cayenne or hot red pepper flakes

4 cups vegetable broth

3 cups cooked chickpeas

1 (14-ounce) can diced tomatoes; or 2 cups diced fresh

¼ cup raisins (optional)

5 ounces baby spinach, washed

1 cup uncooked whole wheat couscous

In a medium saucepan, add oil and onion and sauté until onion is softened and translucent, about 5 minutes. Add garlic, cinnamon, cumin, paprika, salt, pepper, turmeric, and cayenne. Stir until fragrant, about 30 seconds. Add broth, chickpeas, tomato, and optional raisins. Bring to a boil, reduce heat, cover, and simmer on low for 20 minutes.

After simmering, stir spinach and couscous into the hot broth. Cover and let sit for 5 minutes while couscous absorbs liquid and spinach wilts.

Multicooker variation: Use the sauté function for the onion, garlic, and spices, then add broth, chickpeas, tomatoes, and optional raisins. Switch to the pressure-cook function on high for 10 minutes, followed by a natural release. Open lid, stir in couscous and spinach, replace lid, and let sit for 5 minutes before serving.

MAKE IT YOURSELF

Vegetable Broth (p. 293)
Canned Diced Tomatoes (p. 274)

Beans, Greens, and Barley Soup

A fiber-packed soup that is flexible with different combinations of beans and greens. Try black-eyed peas with collard greens, cannellini beans with kale, or Great Northern beans and Swiss chard or spinach. Add wonderful richness to soups using Parmesan cheese rinds; save them in an airtight container in the freezer and pull out as needed.

SERVES 6

1 tablespoon olive oil

1 onion, diced

1 carrot, diced

1 rib celery, diced

2 cloves garlic, minced

1 teaspoon kosher salt

¼ teaspoon hot red pepper flakes

6 cups vegetable broth or water

1 (14-ounce) can diced tomatoes; or 2 cups diced fresh

½ cup pearl barley or wild rice

¼ cup chopped fresh parsley; or 1½ tablespoons dried

1 teaspoon fresh thyme; or ¼ teaspoon dried

1 rind Parmesan cheese (optional)

1 (8-ounce) bunch dark leafy greens

1½ cups cooked black-eyed peas or white beans

freshly ground black pepper

Heat oil in a large Dutch oven or soup pot over medium-high heat. Add onion, carrot, and celery. Cook for about 5 minutes, until vegetables begin to soften.

Add garlic, salt, and hot red pepper flakes. Stir until fragrant, about 30 seconds.

Add broth, tomatoes, barley, parsley, thyme, and optional Parmesan rind. Bring to a boil, reduce heat to a simmer, cover, and cook for 30 minutes.

Remove and compost stems from greens. Chop leaves. Stir in greens and beans. Cover and continue to simmer for another 10 minutes. If you used a Parmesan rind, remove before serving. Season with freshly ground pepper.

MAKE IT YOURSELF

Vegetable Broth (p. 293)
Canned Diced Tomatoes (p. 274)

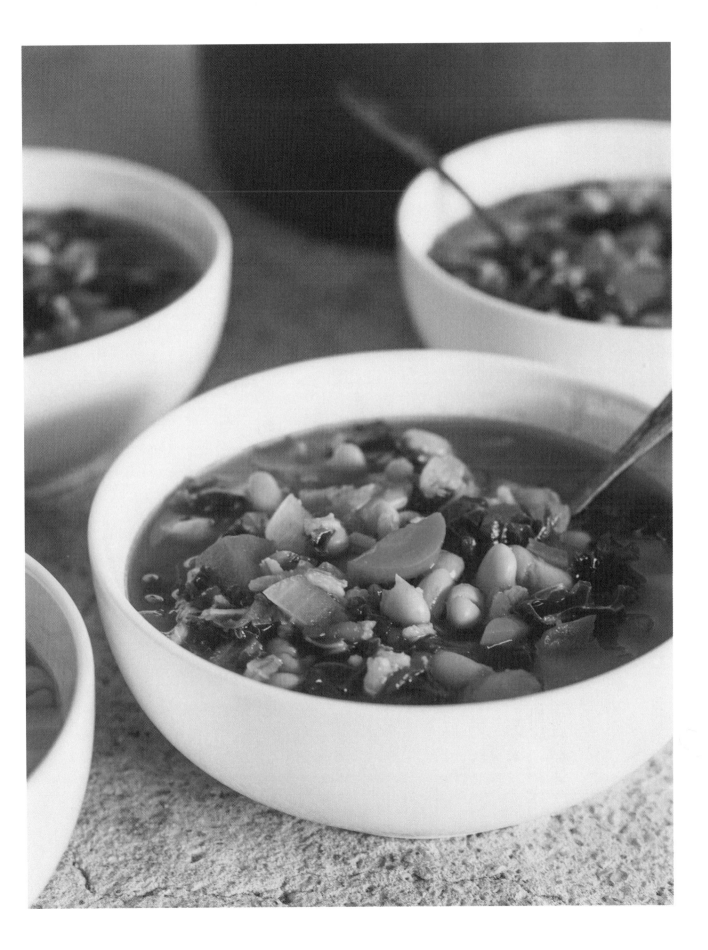

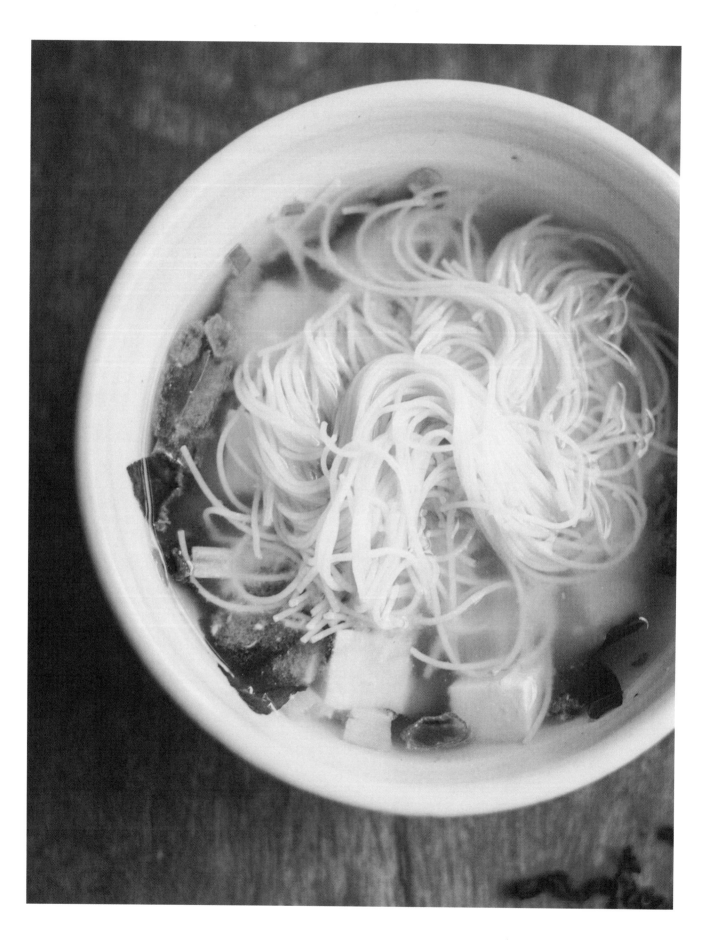

Simple Miso Snack Soup

Soup makes a simple, speedy snack or mealtime appetizer. Adding small tofu cubes to miso broth along with green onions creates a delicious soup in minutes that kids love. Optional seaweed adds nutrients. If you like noodle soups, cooked rice noodles added right before serving work well.

SERVES 6

4 ounces rice noodles (optional)

6 cups water

14 ounces firm tofu, drained and cut into small cubes

2 green onions, finely chopped (both white and green parts)

2 tablespoons ready-to-use dried Wakame seaweed (optional)

6 tablespoons white miso

If using noodles, cook, drain, and rinse under cold water to stop the cooking process. Set aside.

In a soup pot, bring water, tofu, green onions, and optional seaweed to a boil. Turn off heat.

Scoop out about ½ cup hot broth into a small heatproof bowl and add miso. Whisk to combine. Add miso broth to the soup pot and stir. Steep for 1–2 minutes before serving.

If noodles have been prepared, add to individual soup bowls. Top with miso soup.

NOTE: When reheating leftover soup, avoid boiling the miso. Miso is a fermented food containing probiotics (healthy bacteria), which would be killed by boiling.

Split Pea Vegetable Stew

Split peas offer lots of fiber and plant protein at low cost. The flavor base of this recipe is a classic French mirepoix: a trio of onion, carrot, and celery.

SERVES 6

1 tablespoon olive oil

1 onion, chopped

2 carrots, chopped

1 cup chopped celery or celeriac

2 cups split peas or lentils (brown or green), sorted and rinsed

4 cups vegetable broth or water

1 (28-ounce) can crushed or diced tomatoes; or 4 cups diced fresh

3 cloves garlic, finely chopped

1 bay leaf

¼ teaspoon dried thyme

¼ teaspoon kosher salt

¼ teaspoon freshly ground black pepper

OPTIONAL SPICES

1 teaspoon ground cumin

1 teaspoon ground coriander

1 teaspoon ground turmeric

(or 1 tablespoon curry powder)

Heat oil in a soup pot over medium heat. Add onion, carrots, and celery. Cook for 10 minutes, until vegetables are soft and tender. (If Indian flavors are desired, add optional spices at the end of the 10 minutes—either a combination of cumin, coriander, and turmeric or just curry powder.)

Add split peas, vegetable broth, tomatoes, garlic, bay leaf, thyme, salt, and pepper. Bring to a boil. Reduce heat to low, cover, and simmer for 45–60 minutes, or until split peas are tender. (If using lentils, cook for only 45 minutes. *Note:* If your split peas or lentils are old they may take longer to cook.) Stir occasionally.

Remove bay leaf and adjust seasonings to taste, such as additional salt and pepper. As with most soups, flavors improve with time.

MAKE IT YOURSELF

Vegetable Broth (p. 293)
Canned Diced Tomatoes (p. 274)

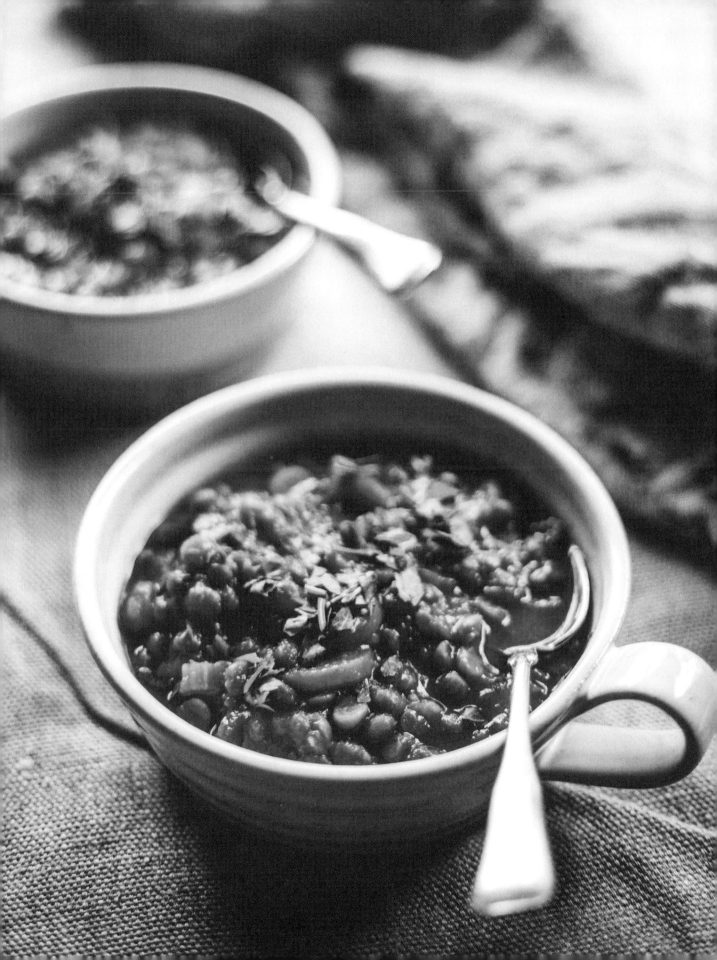

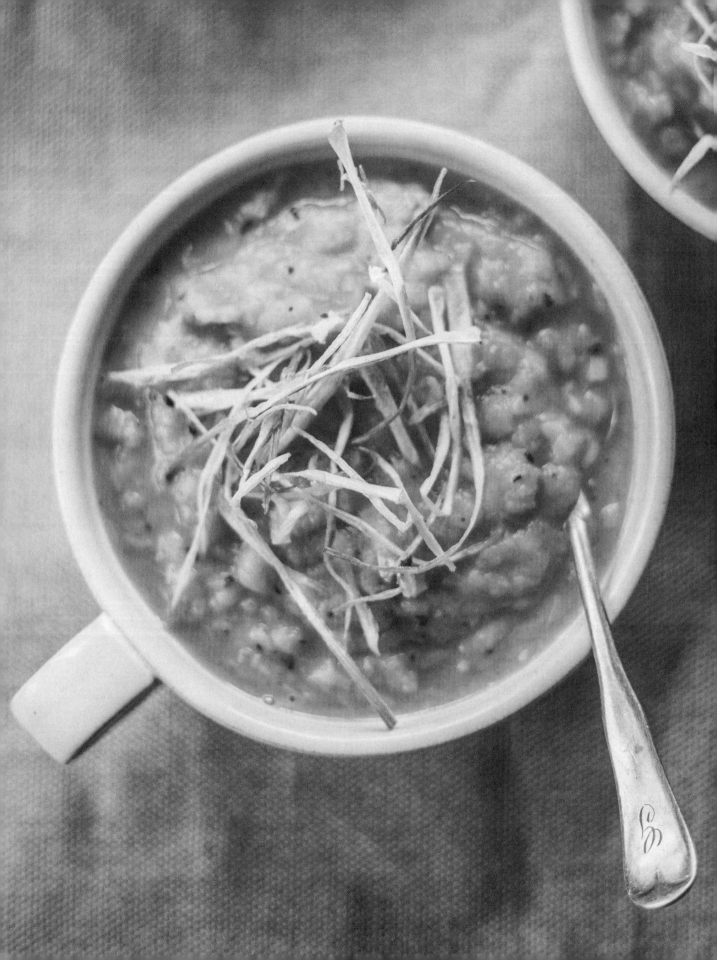

Roasted Butternut Squash Soup

A wonderful soup that uses late-harvest vegetables for days when the weather turns cooler. Roasting the squash and garlic gives depth of flavor to an otherwise simple soup. The optional addition of curry powder will change the flavor profile to a spiced squash soup. The thin skin of butternut squash is edible, so leave on for additional fiber and less food waste. Roast the seeds and use as a garnish or snack.

SERVES 6

Frizzled Leeks (p. 203) for garnish

Roasted Squash Seeds (p. 210) for garnish

1 butternut squash, cut into ¾-inch cubes

2 tablespoons olive oil, divided

kosher salt and freshly ground black pepper

1 garlic bulb (entire head of cloves)

4 cups thinly sliced leek (white and light green parts from about 3 leeks)

1 teaspoon curry powder (optional)

2 cups water

2 cups vegetable broth

NOTE: If you plan to use frizzled leeks as a garnish, prepare those first. Additionally, if you plan to use the butternut squash seeds for a garnish, get them ready first as well so they can go in the oven with the veggies but on a separate baking sheet if you have the room.

In a large bowl, toss cubed squash with 1 tablespoon oil, ½ teaspoon salt, and ½ teaspoon pepper. Spread out squash in a single layer on one or two baking sheets. Place the whole, unpeeled garlic bulb on the sheet as well. Place in a cold oven and turn to 450°F. Start timing and roast for about 30 minutes until squash is tender. If even browning is desired, stir about halfway through the cooking time.

Heat the remaining 1 tablespoon oil in a soup pot over medium heat. Add leeks. Sauté, stirring often, until tender, 7–10 minutes. (For spiced soup, stir in optional curry powder during the final minute of sautéing to bloom the spices.) Remove from heat.

Add water, broth, and roasted squash to the soup pot. Peel the garlic and add the roasted cloves to the pot as well. Puree until smooth using a blender (technique on p. 307).

At serving time, heat soup over medium heat until hot. Season with additional salt and pepper to taste.

Garnish with frizzled leeks, roasted squash seeds, or both, if desired.

MAKE IT YOURSELF

Vegetable Broth (p. 293)

Comforting Cauliflower and Potato Soup

Naturally creamy, cauliflower and potatoes blend together for a comforting cold weather soup. Finishing the soup with a drizzle of extra-virgin olive oil is a must; it lends a rich mouthfeel and robust flavor to the soup.

SERVES 6

¾ cup Crispy Roasted Chickpeas (p. 209) for garnish

2 tablespoons olive oil

1 onion, chopped

3 cloves garlic, minced

kosher salt and freshly ground black pepper

4 cups vegetable broth

1 large head cauliflower, chopped (florets and stem)

4 large Yukon Gold potatoes (about 2 pounds), chopped

½ teaspoon dried thyme

½ teaspoon dried dill weed

extra-virgin olive oil for drizzling

cayenne (optional)

chopped fresh parsley or chives for garnish

If you'd like to garnish this soup with roasted chickpeas, make those first and proceed to the next step while they are roasting.

Heat oil in a large Dutch oven or soup pot. Add onion and sauté for about 5 minutes. Add garlic, 1 teaspoon salt, and ¼ teaspoon pepper and continue cooking for 30–60 seconds. Add vegetable broth, cauliflower, potatoes, thyme, and dill weed. Bring to a boil. Reduce heat, cover, and simmer for 15 minutes, or until potatoes are fork tender.

Remove from heat and blend soup until smooth (technique on p. 307).

Just before serving, drizzle extra-virgin olive oil over top, along with a sprinkle of salt and freshly ground black pepper or cayenne. Garnish with roasted chickpeas and parsley, if desired.

MAKE IT YOURSELF

Vegetable Broth (p. 293)

Tomato Gazpacho

This tasty, refreshing gazpacho is great on those hot summer days when you need to use up garden tomatoes, cucumbers, and peppers!

SERVES 6

3 cups Fresh Salsa (p. 254)

2 cups tomato or vegetable juice

½ cucumber, chopped

½ green bell pepper, chopped

dash black pepper

Prepare a batch of salsa in your food processor. Add tomato juice, cucumber, bell pepper, and black pepper. Process to desired consistency (fine chunks or puree). Refrigerate for at least 2 hours.

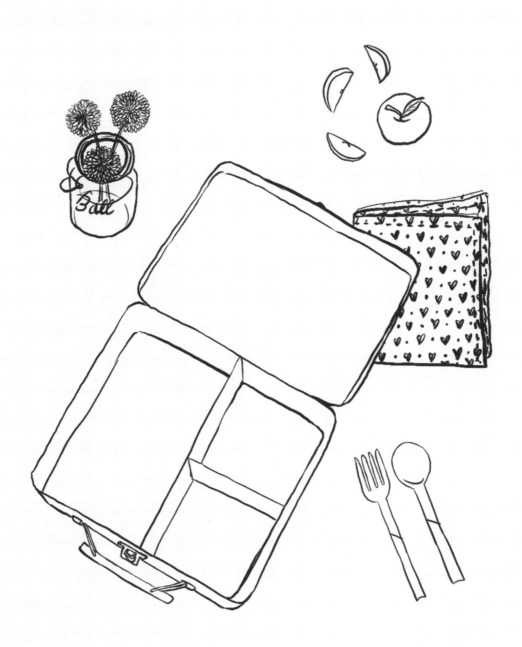

Sandwiches
and Wraps

———

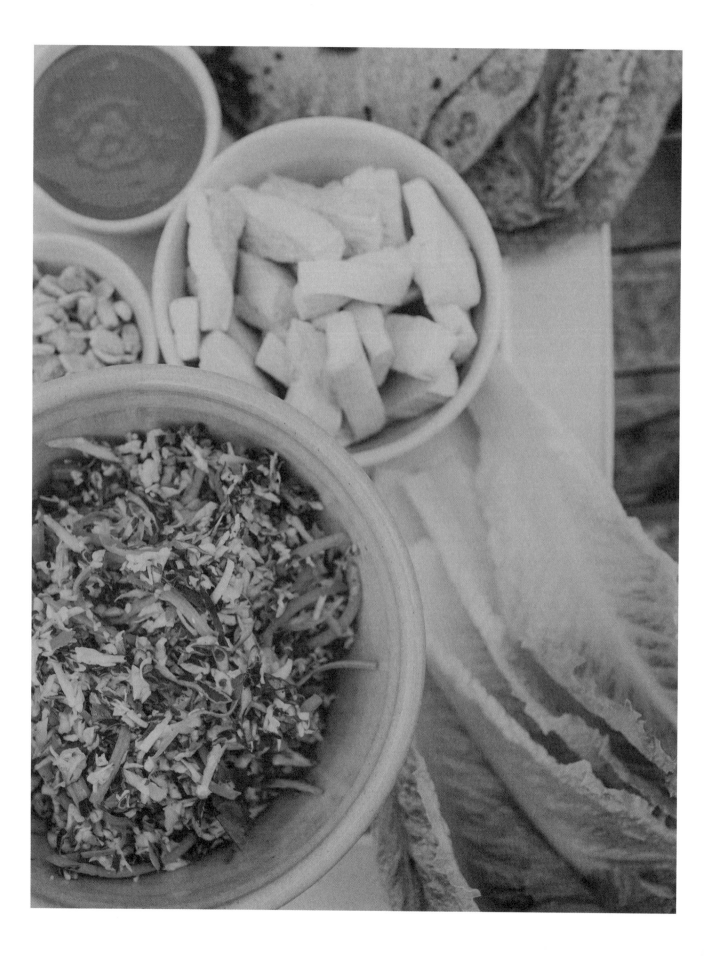

Thai Veggie Tofu Wrap

This refreshing wrap can be made using either whole wheat tortillas or lettuce leaves. The tofu can be used cold in its raw form or sautéed until warmed slightly. For a quickly assembled meal, prepare both the Peanut Sauce and the Cilantro Lime Slaw recipes ahead of time.

SERVES 4

14 ounces firm or extra firm tofu, drained

1 tablespoon canola oil (optional)

4 whole wheat tortillas or large lettuce leaves

½ cup Peanut Sauce (p. 252)

½ cup julienned red bell pepper

½ cup julienned cucumber

¼ cup roasted peanuts

2 cups Cilantro Lime Slaw (p. 201)

Cut tofu into strips. If you prefer to use cooked instead of raw tofu in this wrap, press tofu for at least 20 minutes (technique on p. 311) and then sauté in 1 tablespoon canola oil until golden brown.

Spread 2 tablespoons peanut sauce on each tortilla or lettuce leaf. Divide tofu (raw or cooked) between the tortillas or lettuce leaves. Divide bell pepper, cucumber, and peanuts evenly between the wraps. Top each with ½ cup slaw. Wrap up and enjoy.

MAKE IT YOURSELF

Whole Wheat Tortillas (p. 286)

Caprese Grilled Cheese

Caprese is a simple Italian trio of basil, fresh mozzarella, and tomatoes. The combination just so happens to feature the colors of the Italian flag—green, white, and red—and to be tasty as a sandwich.

SERVES 4

1 tablespoon butter

8 slices sourdough bread

¼ cup Classic Basil Pesto (p. 247)

1-2 tomatoes, sliced and, if using a watery tomato, seeded (8 slices total)

4 ounces fresh mozzarella, sliced or shredded

¼ red onion, thinly sliced

1 avocado, mashed or sliced

Preheat a skillet or griddle over medium heat. The amount of surface area you have will determine how many sandwiches you can grill at a time. Lightly butter each slice of bread on one side, about ¾ teaspoon butter per slice. For each sandwich, spread 1 tablespoon pesto onto one of the bread slices, opposite the buttered side. Place buttered side down on the skillet. On top of the pesto, layer 2 slices tomato, a quarter of the mozzarella, and some onion. Spread the mashed avocado onto the slice of bread that will go on top, on the non-buttered side. Place this slice of bread on top, with the avocado in the sandwich and the buttered side facing up. Cook about 3 minutes, or until the bread is golden brown. Flip with a spatula and cook until the other side is golden brown as well. Repeat for any remaining sandwiches.

MAKE IT YOURSELF

Butter (p. 282)

Antipasto Platter or Sandwich

An Italian word meaning "first course," antipasto is a beautiful plate of ingredients that can easily be adapted as a vegetarian form. These ingredients could be stuffed into or piled on top of a pita to create a sandwich if desired.

SERVES 4

4 (6-inch) whole wheat pitas, sliced into halves

1 cup Classic or Roasted Red Pepper Hummus (p. 251)

1 cucumber, sliced

20 pitted kalamata olives

¾ cup sliced roasted red peppers

4 canned artichoke hearts, quartered

½ cup sun-dried tomatoes; or 1 small fresh tomato, sliced

4 ounces feta, crumbled

chopped fresh parsley, olive oil, and salt and pepper for garnish

Arrange pita, hummus, vegetables, and feta cheese on a platter. Garnish with parsley, a drizzle of olive oil, and salt and pepper. Serve as an appetizer or create a sandwich by stuffing half pita pockets with any or all ingredients.

MAKE IT YOURSELF

Roasted Red Peppers (p. 275)

Loaded Veggie Sandwich with Garlic Herb Spread

"Loaded" is not an understatement here. Your mouth and eyes will be wide with the variety of vibrant vegetables. Serve with a high-protein side such as Edamame Caprese Salad (p. 84) and you've got a well-balanced meal. You can also use the garlic herb spread on a breakfast bagel or as a dip for veggies or crackers.

SERVES 4

GARLIC HERB SPREAD

4 ounces cream cheese, softened, or Lebanese Labneh (p. 228)

1 teaspoon minced garlic

1 tablespoon minced fresh tarragon; or 1 teaspoon dried

1½ teaspoons minced fresh oregano; or ½ teaspoon dried

1½ teaspoons minced fresh basil; or ½ teaspoon dried

SANDWICH

8 slices large sandwich bread

1 cup sprouts or watercress

1 cup salad greens (such as arugula, spinach, baby kale), washed and dried

1 small cucumber, thinly sliced lengthwise

1 avocado, mashed

1 yellow bell pepper, sliced

1 large carrot, thinly sliced lengthwise

1 tomato, sliced

4 radishes, sliced

4 round slices red cabbage, about ¼ inch thick

salt and pepper

Prepare the garlic herb spread: Add cream cheese (or labneh), garlic, tarragon, oregano, and basil to a small bowl. Mix until combined and set aside.

Lay bread slices out on your kitchen workspace. Spread 1 tablespoon garlic herb spread on each slice. Layer the rest of the ingredients in the order listed above, dividing onto 4 slices of bread and seasoning with salt and pepper to taste. Top with the remaining slices of bread. You can either cut sandwiches in half and serve at this point or wrap them in parchment paper and then cut to help hold the sandwich together.

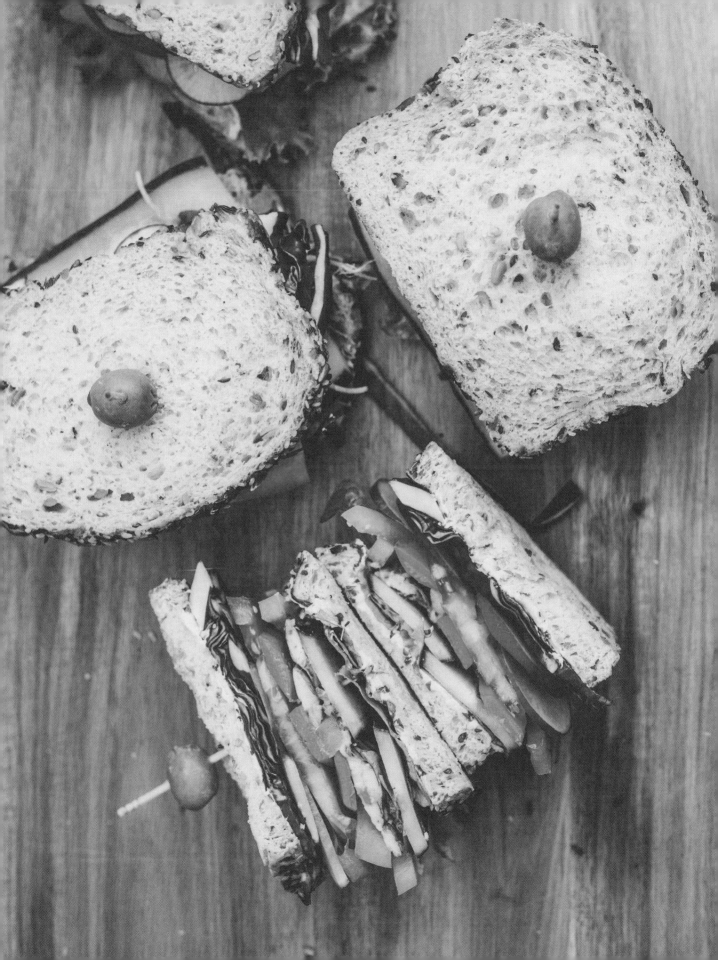

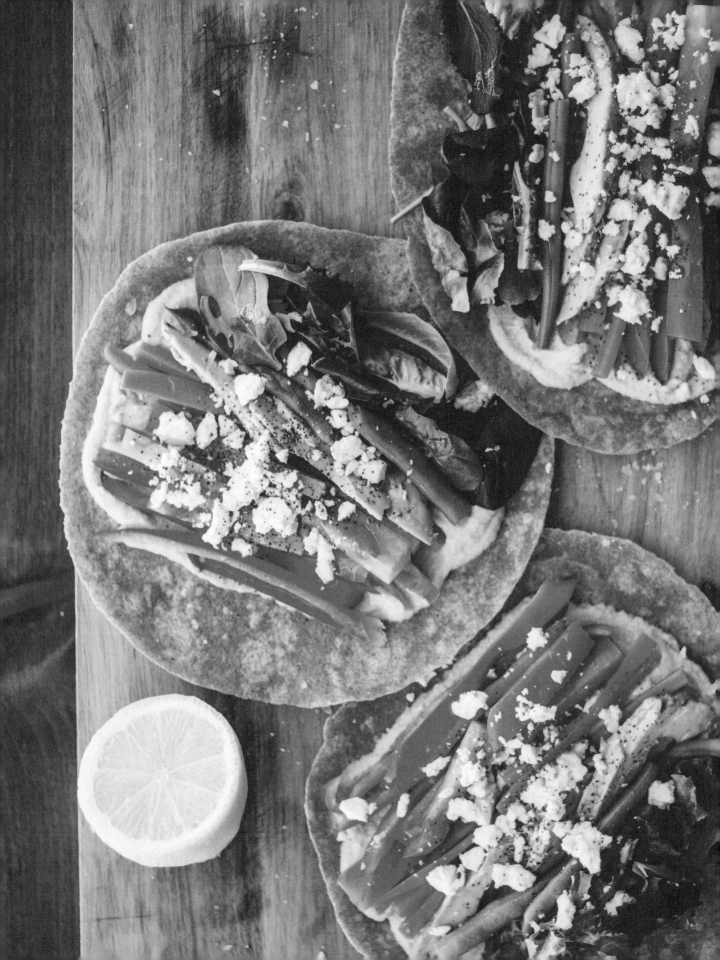

Crunchy Hummus Veggie Wrap

This wrap is a good way to eat a wide variety of raw vegetables in a form other than salad. It is easily adaptable to your favorite veggies or those you have on hand.

SERVES 6

1½ cups Classic Hummus (p. 251)

6 whole wheat tortillas

1 medium carrot, sliced into 2- to 3-inch strips

1 red bell pepper, sliced

2 tomatoes, sliced

3 dill pickles, sliced into 2- to 3-inch strips; or 18 dilly beans

1 avocado, sliced (optional)

2-4 ounces salad greens, washed and dried

1-2 teaspoons extra-virgin olive oil for drizzling

2 ounces feta cheese, crumbled (about ½ cup)

kosher salt and freshly ground black pepper

Spread ¼ cup hummus on each tortilla. Divide the prepared veggies between the 6 tortillas. Drizzle with a little oil and sprinkle on feta cheese and salt and pepper to taste. Wrap up and enjoy.

MAKE IT YOURSELF

Whole Wheat Tortillas (p. 286)
Dilly Beans (p. 276)

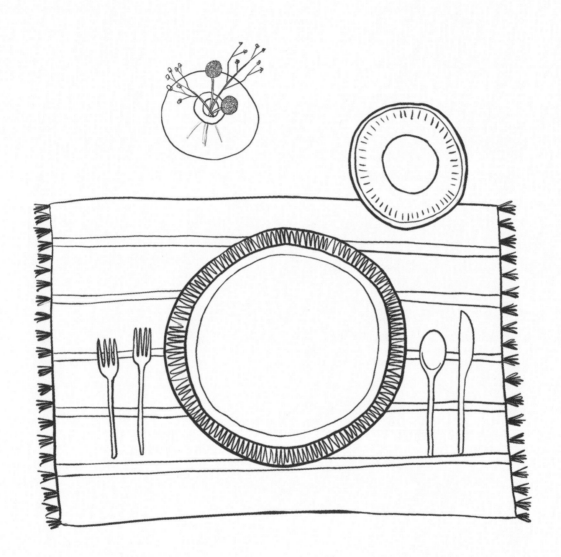

Main Dishes

MODERATION

We are a family of flexitarians. Fish is a regular part of our diet, with local trout and sustainably caught tinned fish as staples. At home we rarely cook other meat. When we are guests of others and a meal with meat is served, we may choose to eat it in moderation. We feel strongly that if we are to eat any meat at all, then we need to be fully aware of the process. On occasion the pot gets used for rooster soup. For everyone's well-being, you can't have more than a couple roos in the hen house. Vegetarian meals never taste better to us than after butchering.

Rather than labeling foods as good or bad, or making specific foods off limits entirely, we prefer to think and talk about foods along a spectrum of health. When less healthy food choices present themselves, we ask questions: What else have I eaten today? Is this one worth it, or is there something later in the day that I might prefer to wait for? Am I on track with getting my food groups in? How much do I need to feel satisfied—can a few bites suffice? When I eat, can I do so mindfully, really enjoying every bite?

Whatever it is that we grow, buy, eat, we've made a practice of talking about it. Nutrition education starts early. At the grocery store with my kids, I talk through how I decide what to put in the cart. "These fruit-flavored yogurt cups have colorful packaging and it's easy to grab one, but it makes more trash than if we buy the bigger container which I can reuse, and it's less expensive to buy bulk. The plain has less added sugar than the flavored. We could add our own vanilla and frozen blueberries, and that would be healthier."

Moderation, intention, conversation: These help us find our way amid the vast array of food choices that confront us every day.

Portabella Mushroom Burgers

For a satisfying burger, marinate portabellas and then grill, broil, or bake. Top with sautéed spinach and caramelized onions to make it special. Serve sweet potato fries alongside, and you've got a great meal.

SERVES 4

4 portabella mushrooms

2 tablespoons olive oil plus additional for rubbing

¼ cup balsamic vinegar

1 tablespoon minced garlic

1 teaspoon kosher salt

½ teaspoon dried basil

½ teaspoon dried oregano

4 whole wheat rolls, sliced, toasted if desired

OPTIONAL TOPPINGS

½ cup Caramelized Onions (p. 202)

4 ounces baby spinach, wilted; or 1 recipe Spinach and White Bean Sauté (p. 186)

roasted red peppers

goat cheese

Prepare any or all optional toppings of your choice.

Remove and compost mushroom stems. Clean off any dirt with a damp cloth. Rub a little oil on the smooth cap of the portabellas. Place them on a baking sheet, with the smooth side of the cap facedown and the gills facing up. Whisk together the balsamic vinegar, 2 tablespoons oil, garlic, salt, basil, and oregano. Pour this marinade onto each of the caps, distributing equally. Let sit at room temperature for 15–30 minutes. Cook mushrooms per your method of choice (see below). Mushrooms are done when fork tender (a fork can easily pierce them).

Grill or Broil on high for 3-5 minutes per side.

Bake: at 400°F (no preheat needed) for about 20 minutes.

Build your burger as desired with our suggested toppings or your own favorites.

MAKE IT YOURSELF

Roasted Red Peppers (p. 275)

Seitan Piccata

Substituting seitan in the more familiar chicken piccata works wonderfully as a meat replacer. This remake uses mostly olive oil with a bit of butter added at the end, improving the nutritional profile while keeping the traditional bright and buttery flavor.

SERVES 4

1 pound Seitan (p. 195)

whole wheat flour for dredging

salt and pepper

2½ tablespoons olive oil, divided

⅓ cup thinly sliced shallots

¼ cup capers, drained

3 cloves garlic, thinly sliced

¼ cup freshly squeezed lemon juice

1 tablespoon butter

Cut seitan chunks in half horizontally so each chunk is now two cutlets. Put flour in a low bowl. Dredge the seitan cutlets so they are covered in flour, but shake off any extra. Sprinkle with salt and pepper.

Add 2 tablespoons oil to a large skillet over medium-high heat. Add seitan cutlets and cook until starting to brown, about 5 minutes. Flip and cook until the other side is also browned lightly. Remove from skillet.

Add remaining ½ tablespoon oil and shallots to skillet and cook over medium heat for about 3 minutes until shallots are beginning to soften. Add capers, garlic, lemon juice, and butter. Stir and continue to cook for 1 minute.

Pour lemon caper sauce over seitan and serve.

MAKE IT YOURSELF

Butter (p. 282)

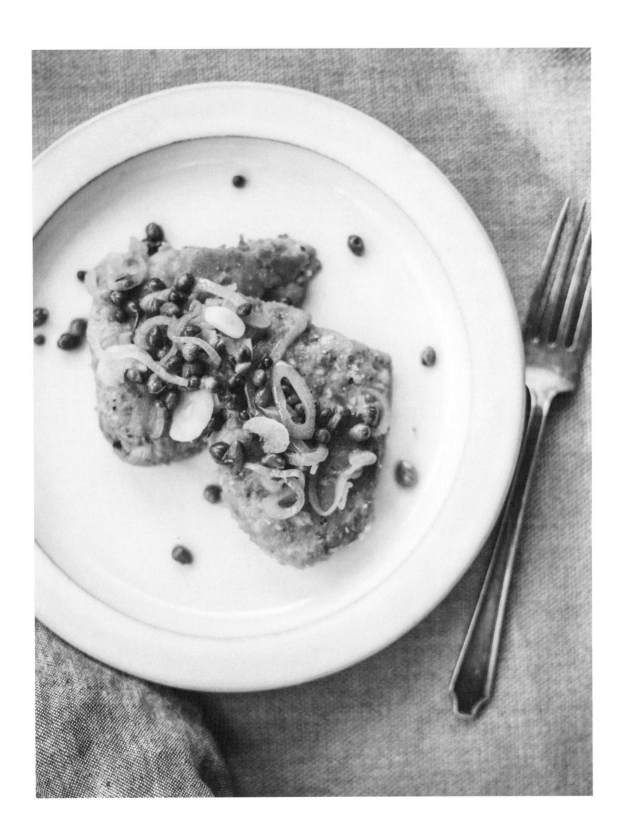

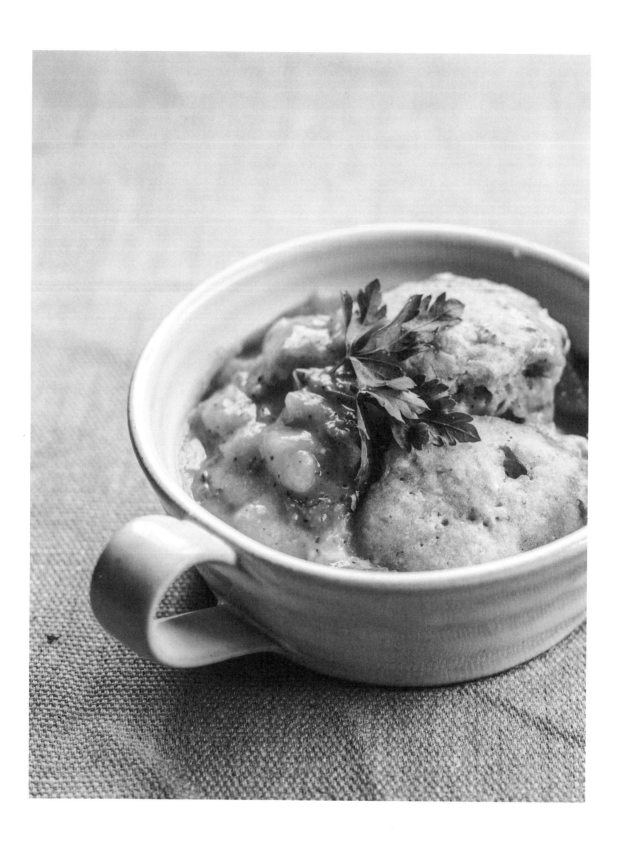

Root Vegetable Potpie with Dumplings

Crowd-pleasing, comforting, creamy food is wonderful in cold weather. This recipe makes use of vegetables that store well through winter months. Cutting vegetables into small, uniform sizes will help them cook evenly and give you several delicious, tender vegetables in each bite.

SERVES 6-8

POTPIE

3 cups vegetable broth

2 cups diced onion

2 cups diced white potato

2 cups diced sweet potato

1 cup diced carrot or parsnip

1 cup diced celeriac or celery

1½ cups milk

½ cup whole wheat flour

¼ cup minced fresh flat-leaf parsley;
or 1½ tablespoons dried

1 tablespoon minced fresh thyme;
or 1 teaspoon dried

1 teaspoon kosher salt

½ teaspoon freshly ground black pepper

1½ cups cooked cannellini beans

1½ cups fresh or frozen peas

WHOLE GRAIN DUMPLINGS

2 cups (234 grams) whole spelt flour
or white whole wheat (254 grams)

1 tablespoon baking powder

½ teaspoon table salt

3 tablespoons cold unsalted butter;
or 2 tablespoons olive oil

¾ cup milk

MAKE IT YOURSELF

Vegetable Broth (p. 293)
Butter (p. 282)

In a large Dutch oven or heavy-bottomed pot with a tight-fitting lid, add broth, onion, white potatoes, sweet potatoes, carrot, and celeriac. Cover, bring to a boil over high heat, then reduce heat and simmer for 10 minutes. In a small bowl, whisk together milk, flour, parsley, thyme, kosher salt, and pepper. Whisk milk mixture into the pot. Stir in beans and peas. Return to a simmer and cook for about 5 minutes more, stirring often, until the broth is thickened.

During the 5-minute simmer, prepare the dough for your dumplings. Measure the flour (technique on p. 310–311). Whisk together flour, baking powder, and table salt. Cut in cold butter (or mix in oil) until the mixture resembles bread crumbs. You can use a fork, pastry cutter, or food processor to cut in the butter. Add milk and stir just enough to combine all the ingredients. Too much stirring will result in a tough dough.

Make sure the broth is bubbling before adding the dumpling dough. Scoop out 1 heaping tablespoon of dough and drop on top of the broth and vegetables. There will be about 16 dumplings in total. Cover the pot tightly and continue to cook over very low heat, barely simmering, for about 25 minutes. Resist peeking; you are using your pot like an oven to capture the heat to cook the dumplings. The dumplings are done when springy to the touch.

Crispy Tofu Parmesan with Sautéed Mushrooms

Tofu can be encrusted and baked crispy in the oven. Serve over spaghetti squash with marinara and top with mozzarella and mushrooms, and you've got a mouthwatering meatless meal. To save time on this multi-recipe dish, you can make the sautéed mushrooms, homemade marinara sauce, and roasted squash ahead of time.

SERVES 4

---

14 ounces extra-firm tofu, drained, or 1 pound Seitan (p. 195)

1 medium spaghetti squash

1 tablespoon olive oil plus additional for drizzling

kosher salt and freshly ground black pepper

2 tablespoons cornstarch

1 egg

½ cup bread crumbs

¼ cup freshly shredded Parmesan cheese

½ cup shredded mozzarella cheese

3 cups (24 ounces) Marinara Sauce (p. 244)

2 cups Sautéed Mushrooms Marinated in Garlic (p. 204; optional but recommended)

MAKE IT YOURSELF

Whole Wheat Bread Crumbs (p. 291)

Press tofu for at least 20 minutes (technique on p. 311).

Cut spaghetti squash in half, remove seeds (clean and roast seeds if desired; see p. 312). Drizzle a little oil on the flesh and sprinkle with salt and pepper to taste. Place on a baking sheet, cut side down. Place in a cold oven and turn to 450°F. Start timing and bake for 35–40 minutes, or until tender. A fork should easily pierce the squash's skin and the flesh will separate easily into strands that resemble spaghetti.

While the squash is roasting, slice pressed tofu lengthwise into 4 slices of even thickness, making rectangular cutlets (slabs about ½ x 2 x 4 inches in size). If using seitan, slice each chunk into two cutlets by cutting them in half horizontally.

Set out three shallow bowls. In one, whisk together cornstarch, ¼ teaspoon salt, and ⅛ teaspoon pepper. In the second, whisk the egg. In the third, mix together bread crumbs and Parmesan cheese. Dip the pressed tofu or seitan, one slice at a time, in the cornstarch. Coat on all sides, brushing excess cornstarch back into the dish. Then dredge it all over in egg. Finally, roll in the bread crumbs, turning to coat.

Cook the tofu by baking or frying (see below). Baking takes longer, but if your oven is already on, the pan can go in along with the squash. Frying is faster but absorbs a bit more of the oil.

To bake: Put 1 tablespoon oil onto a baking sheet, using a spatula to spread it around. Place tofu slices in a single layer on the oiled pan. Bake tofu for 20 minutes at 450°F (oven will be already preheated from roasting squash), flipping the slices halfway through the cooking time. After cooking 20 minutes, top each tofu slice with mozzarella cheese and continue to bake just until cheese melts.

To fry: Put 1 tablespoon oil in an oven-safe skillet (such as cast iron or all stainless steel) over medium-high heat. Fry tofu until golden brown, flip, and cook until other side is crisped. Top each tofu slice with mozzarella cheese and place in the hot oven to melt the cheese.

After baking the spaghetti squash, use a fork to gently scrape the flesh away from the skin. Heat marinara sauce and scooped-out squash together in a large saucepan, stirring often, until the squash is coated and warmed through. Divide between four low bowls or plates. Top with baked tofu and sautéed mushrooms, if desired.

Lentil Shepherd's Pie

A traditional Irish dish that is a great go-to when company is coming for dinner. The key is to never skimp on the mashed potatoes.

SERVES 6

1 tablespoon olive oil

1 cup finely diced onion

1 cup finely diced carrots

1 cup finely diced celery or celeriac

kosher salt and freshly ground black pepper

3 cloves garlic, finely chopped

1 cup green lentils, sorted and rinsed

3 cups vegetable broth or water

2 bay leaves

4 sprigs thyme; or ¼ teaspoon dried

1 (4-inch) sprig fresh rosemary; or ¼ teaspoon dried

2 pounds Yukon Gold potatoes (about 5 medium), chopped into 1-inch cubes

½ cup milk

¼ cup butter

3 tablespoons tomato paste

1 cup frozen peas

MAKE IT YOURSELF

Vegetable Broth (p. 293)
Butter (p. 282)

In a large Dutch oven or oven-safe skillet with a lid (so that it can be covered later), heat oil over medium heat. Add the onion, carrots, celery, and a pinch of salt and pepper. Cook for 10 minutes.

Add garlic and stir for about 30 seconds before adding lentils, broth, bay leaves, thyme, and rosemary. Bring to a boil. Reduce heat to low, cover, and simmer for 30–35 minutes, or until lentils are tender and most of the water has been absorbed. Stir occasionally.

While the lentils are cooking, prepare the potatoes. Place potatoes in a medium saucepan and cover potatoes with water by 1 inch. Stir in 1 teaspoon salt. Bring water to a boil. Reduce heat to medium and simmer potatoes until they are fork tender, about 15 minutes.

Drain the water from the potatoes and return them to the saucepan along with the milk and butter. Mash the potatoes to your desired consistency. Season to taste with salt and pepper.

Once lentils are cooked, remove the bay leaves, any thyme sprigs, and the rosemary sprig. Stir in the tomato paste and peas.

If your skillet is not oven-safe, transfer the lentil mixture to a 2- or 3-quart casserole dish. Spread the mashed potatoes over the lentil mixture in an even layer, using a spoon or fork to add texture to the top of the potatoes for browning.

Place in a cold oven and turn to 375°F. Start timing and bake for 35 minutes, or until potatoes are beginning to brown in spots.

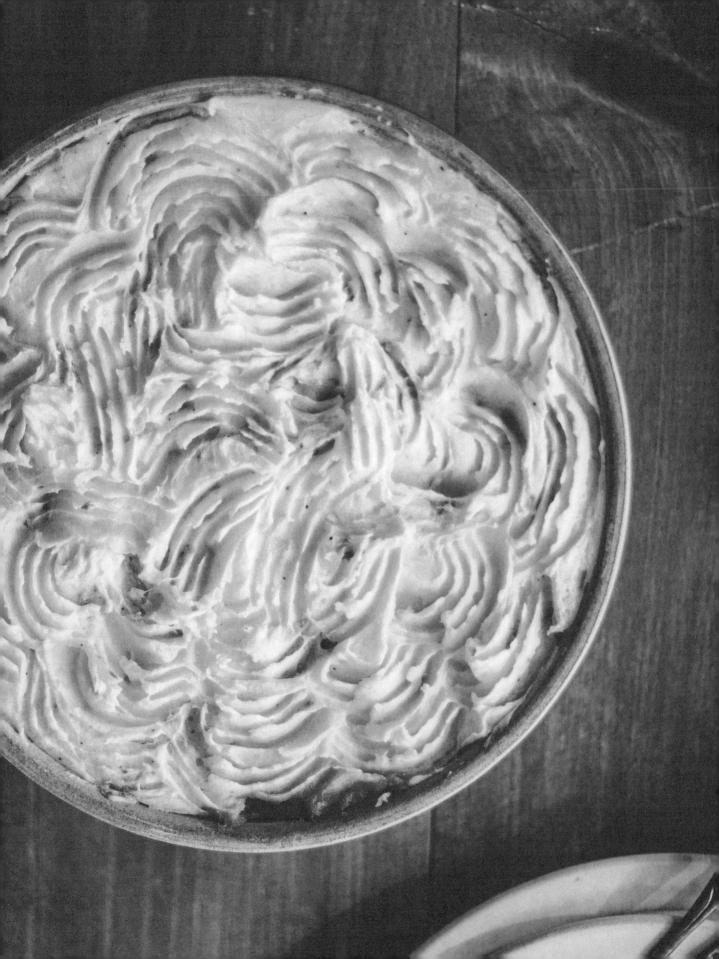

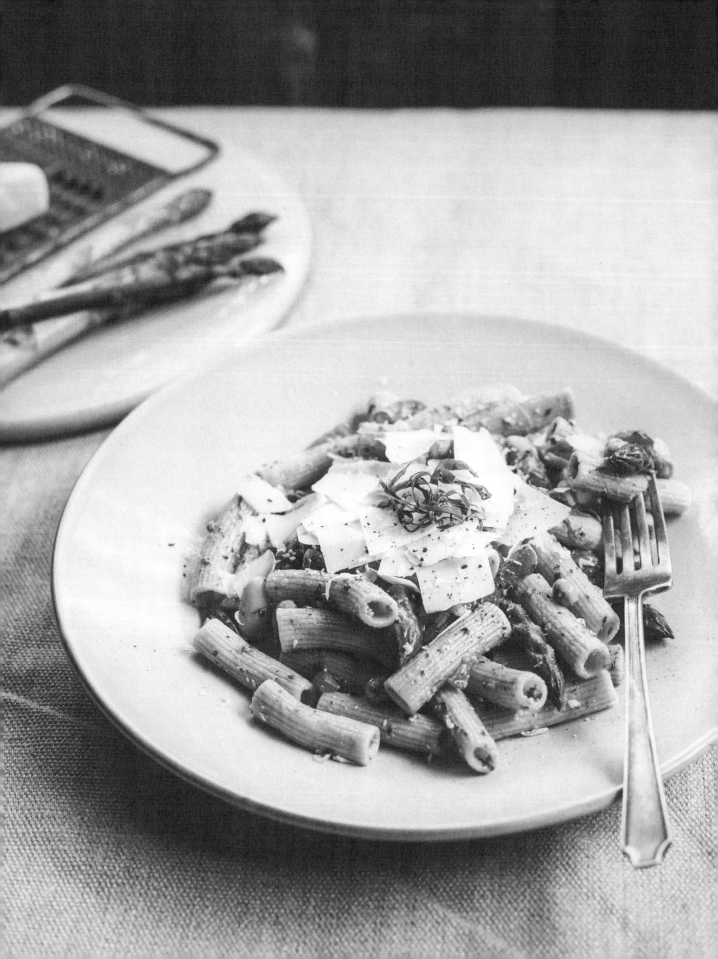

Spring Veggie and Pesto Pasta

Nothing says spring like bright, fresh shades of green. Here we've got asparagus, arugula, peas, and pesto, the first tastes of the season. Serve warm or as a cool salad.

SERVES 4

8 ounces pasta, any variety

1 (8-ounce) bunch asparagus, trimmed and cut into 1-inch pieces (about 2 cups)

½ cup fresh or frozen peas

1½ cups cooked cannellini beans

½ cup chopped roasted red peppers

½ cup Classic Basil Pesto (p. 247)

kosher salt and freshly ground black pepper

freshly grated Parmesan cheese for garnish

a few handfuls arugula (optional)

Cook pasta, setting timer for 3 minutes before pasta will finish cooking. Add asparagus and peas to the pot and boil together for remaining 3 minutes. Drain and return to pot.

Mix in beans, roasted red peppers, and pesto (a pasta fork works well for easy mixing). Stir gently over low heat until beans are warmed and sauce evenly coats the pasta.

Season to taste with salt and pepper and top with freshly grated Parmesan cheese.

If desired, add extra spring green by serving with a handful of arugula either over the top or as a bed underneath.

MAKE IT YOURSELF

Fresh Pasta (p. 289–290)
Roasted Red Peppers (p. 275)

Pumpkin Parmesan Sage Pasta

Imagine how delicious squash-filled raviolis would taste—and how long they would take to make! Create that same taste easily at home by making a pumpkin sauce for your pasta of choice.

SERVES 4

8 ounces fettuccine or other pasta

2 tablespoons olive oil, divided

3 cloves garlic, minced, divided

½ cup chopped walnuts

1½ tablespoons chopped fresh sage

2 cups plain pumpkin puree or pureed winter squash

1 cup fresh or frozen peas

½ cup freshly grated Parmesan or crumbled Gorgonzola cheese

½ teaspoon kosher salt

¼ teaspoon freshly ground black pepper

½–1 cup water, reserved from cooking pasta, or vegetable broth or water

GARNISHES

thickly shaved Parmesan or crumbled Gorgonzola cheese

chopped fresh sage

salt and pepper

Cook pasta. Reserve 1 cup of the cooking water. Drain pasta and toss with 1 tablespoon oil and 1 clove minced garlic. Set aside.

Toast the nuts (technique on p. 312). Set aside.

Heat the remaining 1 tablespoon oil in a skillet over medium heat. Sauté the remaining 2 cloves minced garlic and sage until fragrant, no more than 1 minute. Add pumpkin puree, peas, Parmesan cheese, salt, and pepper. Add water, starting with ½ cup reserved cooking water and adding more if a thinner sauce is desired. Stir and continue cooking until sauce is heated and peas are warmed through. Add the pasta to the sauce and stir to coat (a pasta fork works well for easy mixing). Top with toasted walnuts. Garnish, as desired, with additional cheese, sage, and salt and pepper.

MAKE IT YOURSELF

Fresh Pasta (p. 289–290)

COMMUNITY-SUPPORTED AGRICULTURE

When my husband began studying at Princeton Theological Seminary, we joined a lovely community of people: seminary students and their families in a similar life stage as us. We heard about a few local farms offering shares for a CSA (community-supported agriculture). I had never heard of a CSA until then. We signed up, and I found that I loved getting my big box of seasonal veggies and fruit each week. I relished the challenge of figuring out something to cook with six Japanese eggplants one week and kale that could feed five thousand the next. During art school, I learned that boundaries actually help the creative process. Limits can act as a launching pad for ideas. The same proved true for me with cooking. A CSA was such a great fit because I loved the creativity that is nurtured within the boundaries of seasonal and local.

Jaymie

Veggie Layered Lasagna

Vegetable "noodles" alternate with traditional lasagna noodles, along with layers of tomato sauce and dark green leafy filling, to create one veggie-packed pan! This will feed a crowd or give you leftovers for the week.

SERVES 8

3 cups (24 ounces) Marinara Sauce (p. 244)

8 ounces lasagna noodles (about 10-12)

2 medium eggplants or zucchini; or 1 of each

kosher salt and freshly ground black pepper

¼ cup olive oil, divided

1 pound fresh spinach, kale, collards, or a mix; or 10 ounces frozen spinach, thawed and drained

1 onion, chopped

2 cloves garlic, minced

14 ounces tofu, drained; or 15 ounces ricotta cheese

1½ cups shredded mozzarella cheese (optional)

½ cup nutritional yeast or grated Parmesan cheese, divided

MAKE IT YOURSELF

Fresh Pasta (p. 289–290)

Spread 1 cup marinara sauce over the bottom of a 9 x 13-inch baking pan. Reserve the remaining sauce.

Cook the lasagna noodles. Set aside.

Prepare eggplant or zucchini: Trim off a thin vertical slice to create a flat edge (cook or compost trimmings). Proceed to slice lengthwise, about ¼ inch thick, making slices about the size and shape of the lasagna noodles. A medium eggplant or large zucchini will yield about 6 slices each. Spread out slices and sprinkle evenly with ¼ teaspoon salt. Let rest for 15 minutes, allowing the salt to draw water out of the vegetables. Pat dry with a clean kitchen towel or paper towel. Cook per your preference: on the grill or stovetop or in the oven (see below). Before cooking, lightly oil the vegetable slices with about 1 tablespoon oil.

Grill: Preheat to medium-high. Grill about 5 minutes per side.

Stovetop: Heat a griddle or large skillet over medium heat. Cook eggplant or zucchini in batches that accommodate how much room you have. Flip once browned, cooking about 3 minutes per side.

Oven: Place slices on a baking sheet in a cold oven and turn to 400°F. Start timing and bake for 25 minutes, flipping after 10 minutes.

Once slices are tender and beginning to brown, remove from heat and set aside to cool slightly.

Prepare filling: If using fresh spinach or other greens, wash the greens, remove and compost any tough stems, then finely chop. Heat the remaining 3 tablespoons oil in a skillet over medium heat. Add onion and sauté for about 5 minutes until tender. Add garlic and sauté for another 30–60 seconds. Add chopped greens, ¾ teaspoon salt, and ½ teaspoon pepper. Continue to cook until greens are wilted, about 5 minutes. Remove from heat and set aside.

If using tofu, pulse in a food processor until the tofu resembles the texture of ricotta or cottage cheese. In a large bowl, mix together tofu (or ricotta), 1 cup mozzarella cheese, if desired, and ¼ cup nutritional yeast (or Parmesan cheese). Add wilted greens and stir until evenly distributed.

Assemble lasagna: In the 9 x 13-inch pan that has 1 cup sauce spread over the bottom, place 4 lasagna noodles. Top noodles with about half the filling. Lay 6 vegetable slices (eggplant, zucchini, or both) on top. Top with another 1 cup sauce, then 3–4 more noodles. Spread the remainder of the filling over the noodles. Top with remaining vegetable slices, then remaining 3–4 noodles, 1 cup sauce, and ½ cup mozzarella, if desired.

Cover the pan. Place in a cold oven (or warm if you've roasted the vegetables) and turn to 400°F. Start timing and bake for about 30 minutes, or until hot and bubbly. Sprinkle top with the remaining ¼ cup nutritional yeast (or Parmesan cheese) when it comes out of the oven. Season with additional salt and pepper as desired.

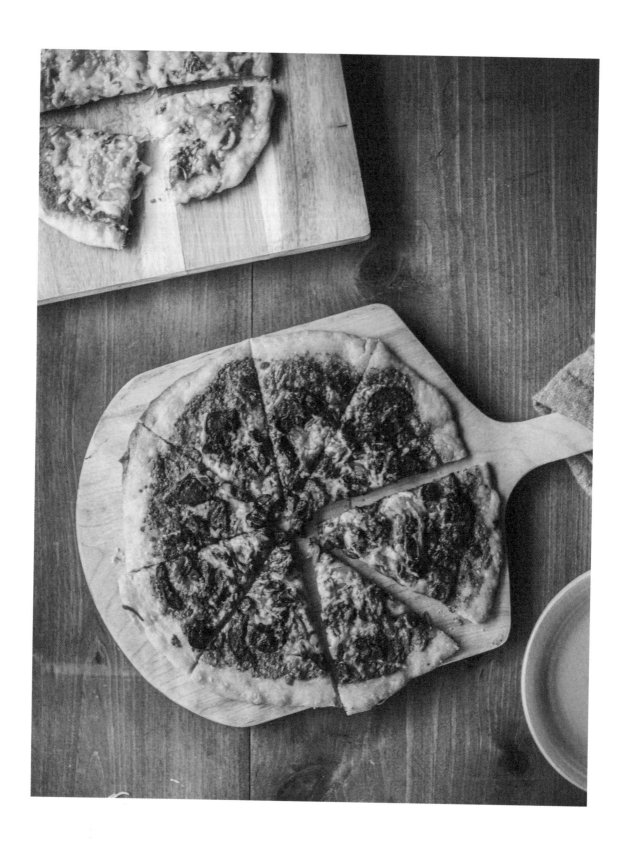

Sprouted Wheat Crust Pizza

This whole grain crust using sprouted wheat (or spelt or white whole wheat) naturally has a sweeter taste than traditional whole wheat. We found sprouted wheat flour from King Arthur Baking Company, an employee-owned B Corp. Start this recipe at least three hours before you plan to eat, to allow the crust fermentation time, which develops flavor. For the tastiest crust, plan for an overnight slow rise in the refrigerator.

SERVES 4

CRUST

2 cups (222 grams) sprouted wheat flour, spelt flour (234 grams), or white whole wheat flour (254 grams)

1 cup (123 grams) all-purpose flour

1¼ teaspoons table salt

¾ teaspoon instant yeast

1¼ cups room temperature or lukewarm water

2 tablespoons extra-virgin olive oil

TOPPINGS

½ cup sauce, such as Classic Basil Pesto (p. 247) or Marinara Sauce (p. 244)

2 cups shredded cheese, such as mozzarella, cheddar, or a combination

toppings of your choice, such as Sautéed Mushrooms Marinated in Garlic (p. 204) or Caramelized Onions (p. 202)

Mixing: Measure the flours (technique on p. 310–311). Whisk together flours, salt, and yeast in a large bowl. Add water and oil. Stir by hand or use a stand mixer with dough hook for about 2 minutes. (Alternatively, put all dough ingredients into a bread machine to mix the dough and complete the first rise, using the dough cycle setting; however, crust will not be as flavorful or light.) The dough will be wet and sticky, as whole grain flours need time to absorb water. Transfer dough to a well-oiled bowl and roll it around so dough is thoroughly coated with oil (an oiled, pliable bench scraper works well if you have one). Cover.

First rise: A full (2 hour) rise at room temperature will about double the dough size. A slow (8-24 hour) rise in the refrigerator yields the best crust results as fermentation develops the flavor. Bring refrigerated dough out about 1½ hours before you plan to bake it. This will allow it 20 minutes to return to room temperature in time for the second rise.

Second rise: Divide dough into balls according to desired pizza size: four balls for personal pan pizzas, two balls for two medium pizzas that can be shared, or one ball for a large family-size

(continued next page)

pizza. Lightly oil a baking sheet. (Alternatively, line the sheet with eco-friendly parchment paper. You will still need to lightly oil the paper). If you have a baking stone, use parchment paper so that it can go directly and easily onto the stone. Pre-shape the dough into thick discs (you'll further stretch them out after the second rise), coat with oil if needed, and place on prepared baking pans. Cover. Allow to rest for 1 hour at room temperature. Dough given plenty of rise time allows the process of fermentation to develop a flavorful crust that is worth the wait.

Topping and baking: Preheat oven to 475°F. Stretch the dough carefully. With oiled fingers, press the discs of dough into flat rounds. Gently pull the edges outward, a little at a time, working your way around the circle. Stretch to the size you desire. Any holes that appear can be gently patched.

Top with sauce, cheese, and vegetables. Bake for about 10 minutes, or until golden brown.

Red Beans and Rice with Kale

Simmering soaked beans in a broth of vegetables, herbs, and spices imparts wonderful flavor that you cannot get when starting from canned beans. Flavor will continue to develop over time, so make this ahead if time allows. Smoked paprika, also known as Spanish paprika, is nice in this dish, if available.

SERVES 8

1 pound (2 cups) dried red kidney beans

1 (8-ounce) bunch kale

2 tablespoons olive oil

1 large onion, chopped

1 large green bell pepper, chopped

3 ribs celery, chopped

4 cloves garlic, minced

5 cups (40 ounces) water, vegetable broth, or a combination

2 teaspoons paprika

1 teaspoon dried oregano

1 teaspoon kosher salt

½ teaspoon freshly ground black pepper

¼ teaspoon hot red pepper flakes

2 bay leaves

½ cup chopped fresh parsley

1 cup uncooked long grain brown rice

1 bunch green onions, thinly chopped, for garnish

MAKE IT YOURSELF

Vegetable Broth (p. 293)

Soak dry beans per method of your choice (technique on p. 313). Drain and rinse the soaked beans. Set aside. Remove and compost kale stems. Chop or tear leaves into bite-sized pieces. Set aside.

In a large Dutch oven or heavy-bottomed pot with a lid (so it can be covered later), heat oil over medium heat. Add onion, bell pepper, and celery. Cook until soft, about 5 minutes, stirring occasionally. Add garlic and cook 1 minute.

Add water, soaked red beans, chopped kale, paprika, oregano, salt, black pepper, hot red pepper flakes, and bay leaves. Bring everything to a boil, then reduce heat to low and cover the pot. Simmer gently for 1½–2 hours until beans are soft. Stir every 30 minutes. The beans should always be just covered by liquid while cooking, so check periodically during cooking and add a bit more water if needed.

When beans are tender, remove from heat. Remove bay leaves and stir in parsley. If you like a creamier texture, remove 1 cup beans and mash with a fork or blend in a food processor, then stir back into the pot.

While the beans are simmering, cook the rice (technique on p. 309).

Serve red beans over cooked rice or mix rice and beans together. Garnish with green onions if desired.

Falafel-Stuffed Pita Pockets

A traditional Middle Eastern food with origins in Egypt, falafel are spiced, mashed chickpeas that have been formed into balls or patties and fried. Start this recipe at least an hour before serving, as the dough should sit in the refrigerator for best flavor and consistency. You can use either fully cooked chickpeas or ones that have only been soaked. Cooked chickpeas will result in a softer falafel, which we prefer. We flatten the falafel in order to use less oil.

SERVES 4

FALAFEL

1½ cups cooked (or soaked) chickpeas

¾ cup chopped shallot or onion

⅓ packed cup chopped fresh parsley

2 teaspoons minced garlic

2 tablespoons raw sesame seeds

1½ teaspoons ground cumin

¾ teaspoon baking powder

¼ teaspoon kosher salt

¼ teaspoon freshly ground black pepper

¼ cup all-purpose flour

¼ cup canola or other neutral oil, for frying

PITA SANDWICH

4 (6-inch) whole wheat pitas, cut into halves

1½ cups Classic Tzatziki (p. 250)

shredded lettuce

chopped tomatoes

Using a clean kitchen towel, pat the chickpeas dry. In a food processor, place chickpeas, shallot, parsley, garlic, sesame seeds, cumin, baking powder, salt, and pepper. Pulse to combine, using a spatula between pulses to scrape down the sides. Stop when everything is combined but the texture is still crumbly.

Add flour 1 tablespoon at a time, pulsing to combine, and scraping down sides. Continue until all flour has been incorporated. The dough should be dry enough to make a ball without sticking to your hands.

Place the dough in a bowl, cover, and refrigerate for at least 1 hour.

Remove dough from refrigerator. Scoop out 1 heaping tablespoon of dough, form into a ball, then flatten into a disc about 2 inches in diameter. Dough should make about 12 discs.

Heat a large skillet over medium heat. Add about half the oil, 2 tablespoons, to coat the bottom of the skillet. Add 6 falafel. Cook 2–3 minutes on each side, or until golden brown. Remove from the skillet. Add remaining oil to the hot skillet and cook the remaining falafel.

Stuff each pita pocket half with 1½ falafel, tzatziki, shredded lettuce, and chopped tomato. Tahini sauce or hummus (p. 251) could be substituted for or used in addition to the tzatziki. Use leftover falafel within several days, or cool completely and freeze for up to 1 month.

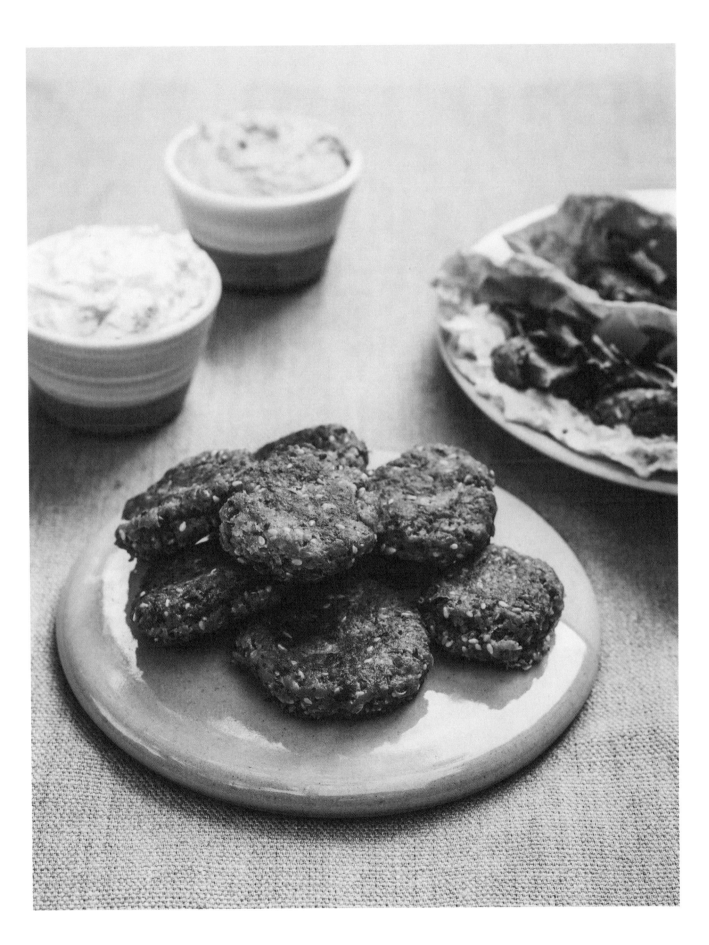

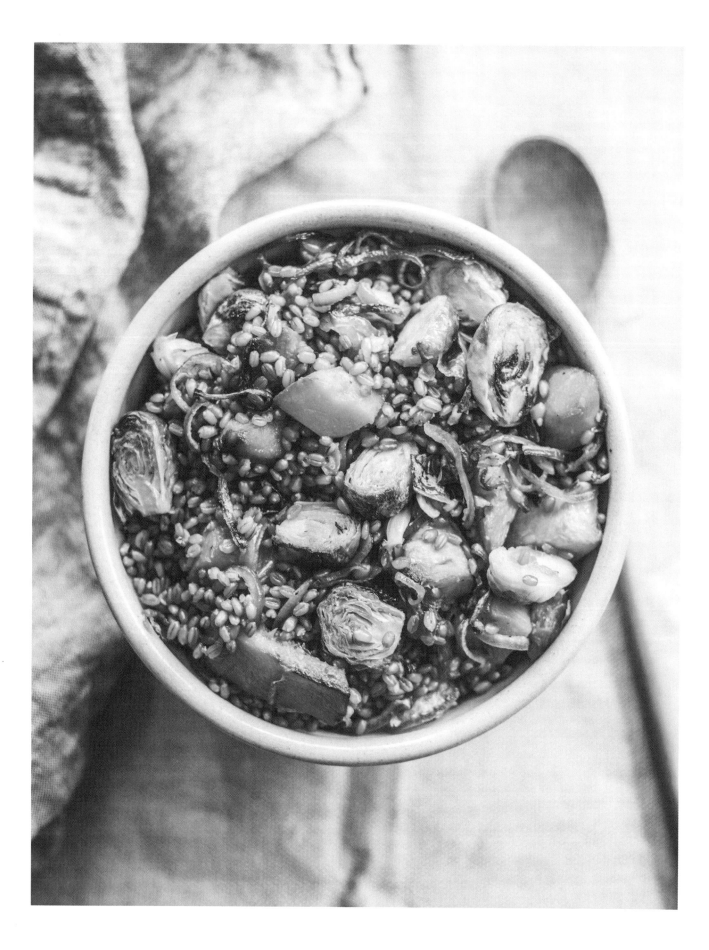

Winter Wheat Berry Bowl
with Agrodolce Sauce

An agrodolce sauce—agro (sour), dolce (sweet)—is an Italian sweet and sour sauce, and it dresses up this hearty whole grain bowl with roasted veggies. Waste not! The thin skin of the butternut squash is edible. Seeds can be roasted for a snack, or they can be used to garnish this recipe. Can't find wheat berries? Substitute another whole grain such as Kamut, spelt, whole oat groats, barley, or brown rice. Cooking times will need to be adjusted for the grain you choose.

SERVES 4

BOWL

3 cups water

1 cup winter wheat berries or another whole grain, sorted and rinsed

1 teaspoon kosher salt, divided

1 butternut squash, cut into ¾-inch cubes (reserve seeds for roasting)

1 pound brussels sprouts, trimmed and halved

1 red onion, thinly sliced

2 tablespoons olive oil

⅛ teaspoon freshly ground black pepper plus additional to taste

toasted walnuts or Roasted Squash Seeds (p. 210) for garnish (optional)

AGRODOLCE SAUCE

⅓ cup red wine vinegar

2 tablespoons honey

1 clove garlic, minced

½ teaspoon hot red pepper flakes

¼ cup extra-virgin olive oil

Put water, wheat berries, and ½ teaspoon salt in a medium saucepan. Bring to a boil. Reduce heat, cover, and simmer for 1 hour, or until tender. (Alternatively, pressure-cook the wheat berries for 30 minutes followed by a 10-minute natural release.) Drain excess water. Set aside to cool.

While wheat berries are cooking, prepare your vegetables. In a large bowl, mix squash, brussels sprouts, onion, oil, pepper, and the remaining ½ teaspoon salt until well coated.

Spread out vegetables in a single layer on two baking sheets. Place in a cold oven and turn to 450°F. Start timing and roast until vegetables are tender and beginning to caramelize, about 30 minutes. If even browning is desired, stir about halfway through the cooking time.

If roasting the squash seeds for a garnish, these can go in the oven with the vegetables on a separate baking sheet if you have the room. Remove seeds after 15 minutes of roasting.

While the vegetables are roasting, prepare the agrodolce sauce. In a small saucepan, simmer red wine vinegar, honey, garlic, and hot red pepper flakes until reduced and syrupy, about 10 minutes on low heat. Stir often. Turn off heat and whisk in oil to complete the sauce.

In a large bowl, mix together cooked wheat berries, roasted veggies, and agrodolce sauce. Toast the nuts (technique on p. 312), if using. Garnish with either toasted nuts or roasted seeds if desired.

Roasted Veggie and Chickpea Bowl

On the basis of their nutrient content, vegetables are categorized into five subgroups: dark green, red and orange, starchy, beans and peas, and other. This one nutrient-packed bowl can get you all five categories!

SERVES 4

1 recipe Zesty Garlic Kale Salad (p. 67)

1½ cups cooked chickpeas

1 sweet potato, diced

2 tablespoons olive oil, divided

1 teaspoon chili powder

½ teaspoon ground cumin

½ teaspoon paprika

¼ cup uncooked quinoa

½ cup water

1 cup julienned raw vegetables, such as carrots, bell peppers, summer squash

Classic Hummus (p. 251)

Prepare kale salad.

Pat chickpeas dry with a clean kitchen towel. Add chickpeas to a small bowl and toss with 1 tablespoon oil and the chili powder. Transfer to one side of a baking sheet in a single layer. Then toss the sweet potatoes in the same bowl with the remaining 1 tablespoon oil, cumin, and paprika. Transfer to the other side of the baking sheet, also in a single layer. Place in cold oven and turn heat to 400°F. Start timing and cook for 30 minutes.

While the sweet potatoes and chickpeas are roasting, cook the quinoa. In a small saucepan, bring quinoa and water to a boil. Reduce heat, cover, and simmer for 15 minutes. Remove from heat and let sit, covered, for another 5–10 minutes. Fluff quinoa with a fork.

Assemble by dividing kale salad evenly between four bowls (about 1 heaping cup in each), then adding roasted chickpeas, sweet potatoes, quinoa, and julienned vegetables. Top with a small scoop of hummus, if desired.

Hearty White Bean Ratatouille

Garlic, herbs, fresh produce, and olive oil create a lovely Mediterranean-style dish. The addition of beans can turn this vegetarian stew into a main meal when served along crusty bread or whole grain pasta. No need to peel your tomatoes or eggplant unless you prefer to do so. This dish tastes best when allowed to sit for a day, so make it ahead if times allows.

SERVES 4

5 tablespoons olive oil, divided

4 cloves garlic, thinly sliced

2 pounds fresh tomatoes, diced; or
1 (28-ounce) can diced or crushed

½ cup chopped fresh parsley

¼ cup chopped fresh basil

1 teaspoon kosher salt, divided

¼ teaspoon freshly ground black pepper

1 medium eggplant, diced (about 5 cups)

1 green bell pepper, diced

1 onion, diced

2 medium zucchini, diced (about 4 cups)

1½ cups cooked cannellini beans

freshly grated or shaved Parmesan cheese, and fresh basil or a dollop of Classic Basil Pesto (p. 247) for garnish

MAKE IT YOURSELF

Canned Diced Tomatoes (p. 274)

In a large Dutch oven or heavy pot with a lid, heat 1 tablespoon olive oil over medium heat. Add garlic and stir for about 30 seconds. Add tomatoes, parsley, basil, ½ teaspoon salt, and black pepper. Cover, reduce heat to low and start simmering the sauce.

Meanwhile, toss diced eggplant with ¼ teaspoon salt in a colander. Set aside. This allows the salt to draw out some of the water in the eggplant. Pat dry with a clean kitchen towel.

Heat a large skillet over medium heat. Add 1 tablespoon oil. Sauté bell pepper, onion, and ⅛ teaspoon salt over medium-low heat, stirring occasionally, until tender, about 10 minutes. Add sautéed peppers and onions to simmering pot of sauce. Return skillet to heat, add zucchini along with another tablespoon oil and ⅛ teaspoon salt. Sauté until tender, about 5 minutes, then add to the simmering pot of sauce.

Add the remaining 2 tablespoons oil and eggplant to the skillet. Cook until tender, about 10 minutes. Add to the sauce. Cover and simmer for an additional 30 minutes. Stir occasionally.

Add beans. Simmer for an additional 10 minutes, or until the beans are warmed through.

Allow to cool slightly before serving (ratatouille is best served warm or at room temperature).

Garnish with Parmesan cheese and basil if desired.

Herby Harvest Bowl
with Toasted Israeli Couscous

Israeli couscous, a type of pasta, is also called pearl couscous, as it is about the size of small pearls. It combines with warm winter squash, sautéed mushrooms, and spinach to create a satisfying grain bowl.

SERVES 4

1 butternut squash, chopped into ¾-inch cubes (no need to remove skin)

3 tablespoons olive oil, divided

1 teaspoon ground sage; or 1 tablespoon minced fresh

kosher salt and freshly ground black pepper

1 cup Israeli couscous

1 large shallot, minced

¼ teaspoon hot red pepper flakes

2 cups vegetable broth; or 1 (14-ounce) can unsweetened coconut milk

1 tablespoon minced fresh parsley; or 1 teaspoon dried

1 tablespoon minced fresh oregano; or 1 teaspoon dried

1 pound cremini (baby bella) mushrooms, washed, trimmed, and sliced

3 cloves garlic, minced

2 teaspoons onion powder

½ teaspoon dried thyme

5-6 ounces fresh spinach, chopped

MAKE IT YOURSELF

Vegetable Broth (p. 293)

Place butternut squash in a bowl with 1 tablespoon oil, sage, ¼ teaspoon salt and ⅛ teaspoon pepper. Mix to evenly coat. Transfer to baking sheet and spread out in a single layer. Place in a cold oven and turn to 450°F. Bake for 30 minutes, or until tender. If even browning is desired, stir halfway through cooking time.

Meanwhile, toast couscous by heating 1 tablespoon oil in a saucepan. Add couscous, shallot, and hot red pepper flakes. Sauté over medium heat until lightly toasted and shallot is tender, about 3 minutes, stirring often. Add broth or coconut milk and bring to a low boil. Cover and simmer for 8 minutes. Be careful not to overcook, as the bottom can burn easily. Remove from heat and allow to sit, covered, for several minutes. Stir in parsley and oregano, then set aside.

Heat the remaining tablespoon of oil in a skillet. Add mushrooms to the pan and sprinkle with ½ teaspoon salt and ⅛ teaspoon pepper. Stir and cook about 3 minutes, over medium-high heat.

Add garlic, onion powder, and thyme to the skillet and stir. Once the garlic is fragrant, after about 30 seconds, add the chopped spinach and stir lightly until wilted.

Combine squash, couscous, and sautéed mushrooms with spinach. Serve warm.

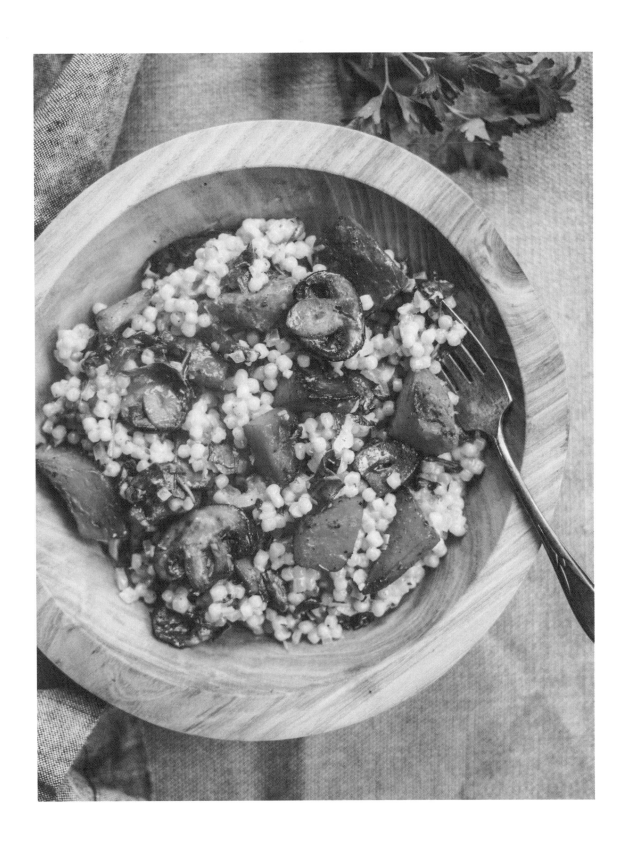

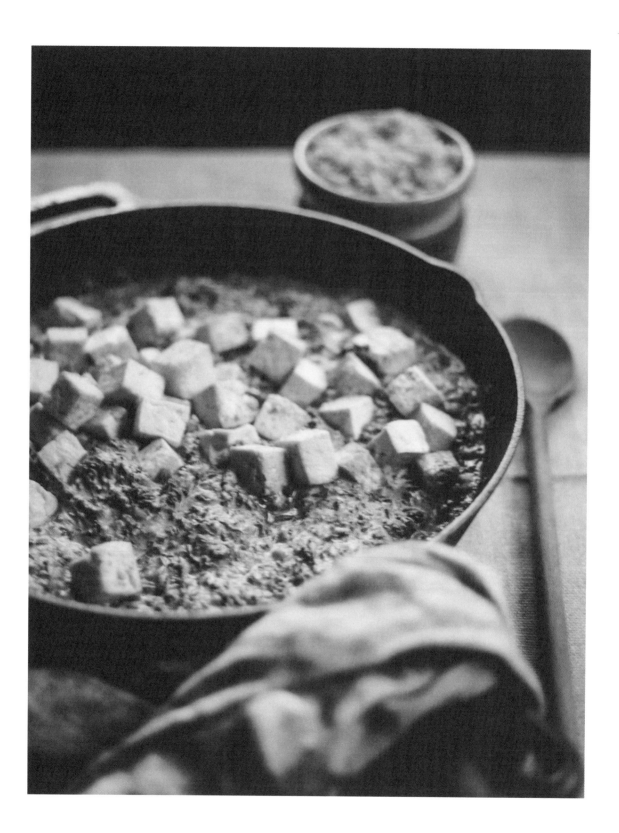

Saag Paneer

A yummy way to get lots and lots of greens. Saag translates to "greens," so you can substitute any greens that cook well—such as kale, chard, collards, or even beet greens—for the spinach in this dish. Feel free to mix a few different kinds to get the full amount! Paneer, an Indian cheese, can be found in international grocery stores. Tofu will substitute well if you aren't able to find it.

SERVES 4

1 cup uncooked brown basmati rice

3 tablespoons canola oil, divided

1 onion, chopped

¾ teaspoons kosher salt, divided

1 teaspoon ground cumin

1 teaspoon ground coriander

1 teaspoon chili powder

1 pound fresh spinach or other dark leafy greens

1 tablespoon grated fresh ginger

1 teaspoon minced garlic

1 chile pepper (serrano or Thai), minced; or ⅛ teaspoon cayenne (optional)

1 (14-ounce) can diced tomatoes; or 2 cups diced fresh

8 ounces paneer cheese, cubed; or 14 ounces firm tofu, drained and cubed

1 (14-ounce) can unsweetened coconut milk

MAKE IT YOURSELF

Canned Diced Tomatoes (p. 274)

Cook rice (technique on p. 309).

Warm 1 tablespoon oil in a large skillet over medium-low heat. Add the onion and ⅛ teaspoon salt. Sauté for about 10 minutes, until onions are very soft. Add the cumin, coriander, and chili powder. Stir for about 1 minute until fragrant. Add the spinach and stir occasionally until wilted. You may need to add several handfuls at a time, allowing them to wilt down. Remove from heat and allow to cool slightly. Add to a food processor and pulse until evenly incorporated. Do not puree. Set aside.

In the same skillet, heat 1 tablespoon oil over medium heat. Add ginger, garlic, and optional chile pepper or cayenne. Sauté for 1 minute. Pour in diced tomatoes, stir and simmer until the mixture starts to darken, about 10 minutes.

While tomatoes are cooking, heat the remaining 1 tablespoon oil in another skillet. Add the cubed paneer (or tofu). Cook until lightly browned, about 10 minutes, stirring occasionally. Remove from heat and set aside.

Add the spinach and onion mixture to the tomato mixture, then pour in the coconut milk. Stir well, then add the paneer (or tofu) and the remaining salt (or to taste). Heat to a light boil.

Serve hot over cooked rice.

Gobi Masala

A vegetarian twist on tikka masala, with gobi (cauliflower) replacing the spicy chicken. This rich and tangy masala sauce has its origins in northern India. The recipe here makes 1½ cups masala paste, but you will use only ¼ cup. Freeze the extra in ¼-cup portions to use later, or if you prefer to store a smaller amount, cut masala paste recipe in half.

SERVES 4

---

1 cup uncooked brown basmati rice

1 cup Raita (p. 253)

fresh cilantro and garam masala for garnish

GOBI

1 head cauliflower, chopped (about 4 cups)

1 tablespoon olive oil

1 teaspoon chili powder

½ teaspoon ground cumin

MASALA PASTE

2 onions, peeled and quartered

5 cloves garlic, peeled and halved

½ packed cup chopped cilantro

¼ cup almonds

2 tablespoons chopped fresh ginger

1 tablespoon freshly squeezed lemon juice

3 tablespoons garam masala

1 tablespoon chili powder

1 tablespoon ground turmeric

1 tablespoon ground cumin

1½ teaspoons ground cloves

½ teaspoon cayenne

2 teaspoons kosher salt

MASALA SAUCE

1 tablespoon olive oil

2 cups tomato puree or 2–3 fresh tomatoes, blended; or 1 (14-ounce) can diced, blended

1 (14-ounce) can unsweetened coconut milk; or 1 cup plain Greek yogurt

Cook the rice (technique on p. 309) and prepare the raita.

Make gobi: Combine all gobi ingredients in a bowl and mix until combined. Transfer to a baking sheet. Place in a cold oven and turn to 450°F. Start timing and bake for 25 minutes. If even browning is desired, stir about halfway through the cooking time.

Make masala paste: Place all masala paste ingredients in a food processor and pulse until it comes together in a paste. Reserve ¼ cup for the sauce and freeze the rest in ¼-cup portions for future meals.

Make masala sauce: Heat the oil in a skillet, then add ¼ cup masala paste. Stir until fragrant, 3–5 minutes. Add the tomato puree and simmer until the sauce is deep red, 5–10 minutes. Stir in the coconut milk and simmer until heated through, not longer.

Add the roasted cauliflower to the sauce and serve hot over brown basmati rice. Garnish with cilantro and a few shakes of garam masala if desired. Serve with raita to cut the spice and boost the protein.

MAKE IT YOURSELF

Canned Diced Tomatoes (p. 274)

Greek Yogurt (p. 280–281)

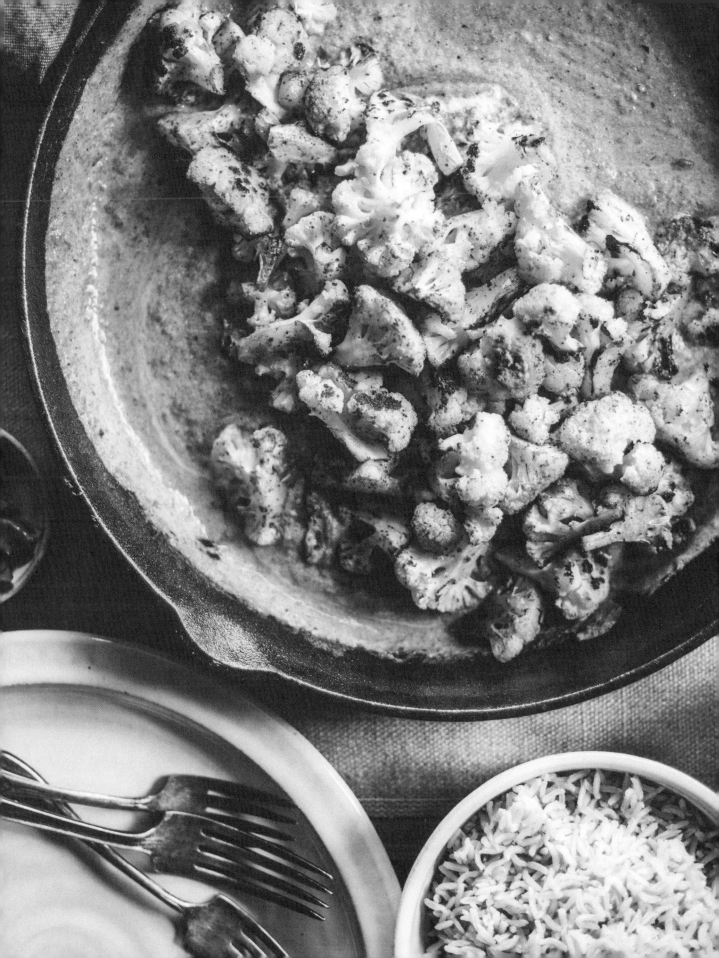

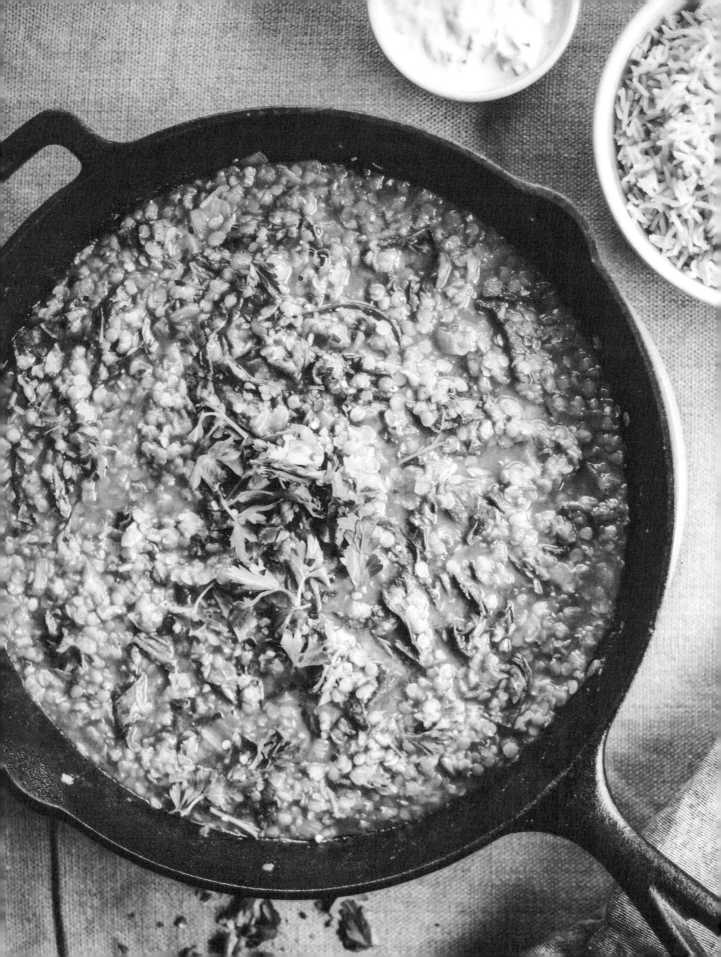

Red Lentil Dhal

In this Indian-style dhal, "blooming" the spices—cooking them briefly in oil—releases fat-soluble flavor compounds. This makes them, by some estimates, ten times more flavorful and allows flavors to be distributed more evenly throughout your dish.

SERVES 4

---

1 cup uncooked brown basmati rice

1 cup Raita (p. 253)

2 tablespoons canola oil

1 onion, chopped

2 teaspoons minced garlic

1 teaspoon grated fresh ginger

2 teaspoons curry powder

1 teaspoon ground cumin

¼ teaspoon hot red pepper flakes

3 cups water

1 cup red lentils, sorted and rinsed

1 medium tomato, chopped

½ teaspoon kosher salt

4 packed cups baby spinach or chopped mature spinach leaves

Cook the rice (technique on p. 309) and prepare the raita.

Heat oil in a medium saucepan. Add onion and sauté over medium heat until tender, about 5 minutes.

Bloom your spices by adding the garlic, ginger, curry powder, cumin, and hot red pepper flakes to the sautéed onion. Cook for 30 seconds, stirring the whole time.

Add water, lentils, tomato, and salt. Bring to a boil, reduce heat to a low simmer, partially cover the saucepan, and cook for about 20 minutes. Stir occasionally. The water should be mostly cooked out of the pot. Remove from heat. Add spinach to the hot dhal and stir until wilted. Serve with rice and raita.

Red Lentil Coconut Curry

This mild curry is great for kids or adults who prefer a lower level of heat. The vegetables you use can flex to match what you have on hand.

SERVES 4

1 cup uncooked brown rice; or Indian bread, such as naan, to serve 4

2 tablespoons canola oil

2 onions, chopped

1 tablespoon curry powder

1 tablespoon minced garlic

1 teaspoon grated fresh ginger

⅛ teaspoon cayenne, or to taste (optional)

3-4 cups water or vegetable broth

1 (14-ounce) can unsweetened coconut milk

1 cup red lentils, sorted and rinsed

2 cups chopped fresh or frozen green beans

2 cups chopped fresh or frozen cauliflower florets

1 cup chopped carrot

1 teaspoon kosher salt

1 bay leaf

½ cup chopped fresh cilantro plus additional for garnish

½ cup cashews or peanuts for garnish

If you plan to serve with rice, cook rice now (technique on p. 309).

Heat oil in a Dutch oven or heavy-bottomed pot with a lid (so that it can be covered later) over medium-low heat. Add onions, stirring often, until starting to brown, about 10 minutes. Add curry powder, garlic, ginger, and optional cayenne. Sauté for 1 minute.

Add water (3 cups for a thicker curry, 4 cups for thinner), coconut milk, lentils, green beans, cauliflower, carrot, salt, and bay leaf. Stir to combine. Bring to a boil over medium-high heat, then reduce heat, partially cover, and simmer for 20 minutes.

Once the curry has finished cooking, remove bay leaf. Stir in ½ cup cilantro. Enjoy as is or puree to desired consistency (technique on p. 307). Garnish with cashews and additional cilantro if desired. Adjust seasonings to taste. Serve over rice or with naan or another bread.

MAKE IT YOURSELF

Vegetable Broth (p. 293)

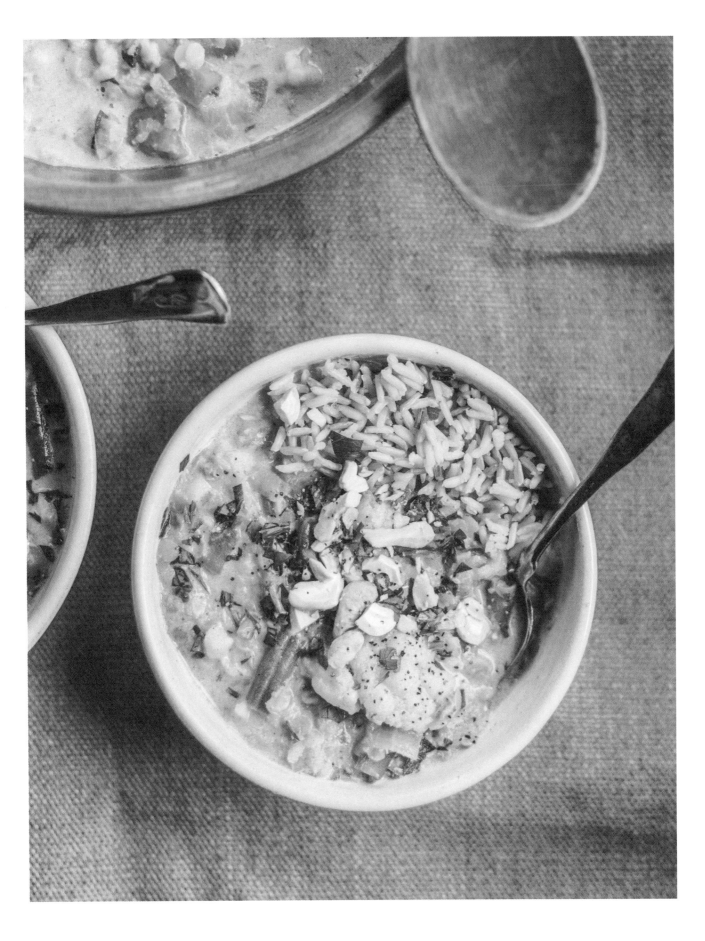

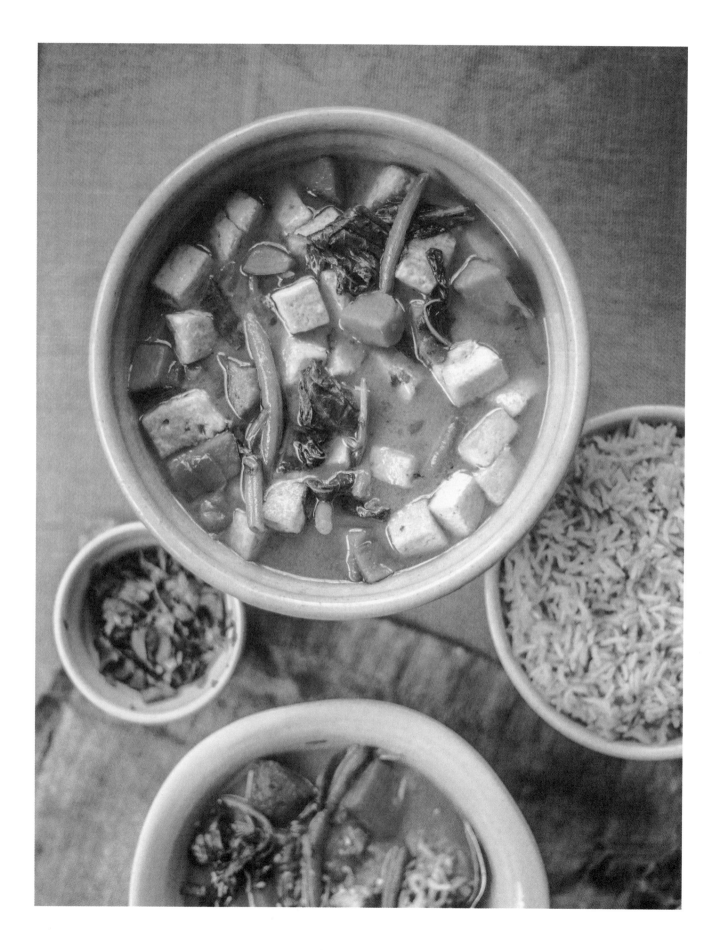

Green Curry Vegetables

This rich, creamy Thai dish manages to be both warm and comforting and fresh and vibrant. The veggies can be swapped out for similar ones you have on hand—for example, carrot instead of sweet potato; broccoli instead of baby kale or spinach. It's a great way to use up what you have. You can find green curry paste in the Asian food section of most grocery stores, usually in a small glass jar next to red curry paste (also delicious, and milder if you prefer less heat).

SERVES 4

1 cup uncooked rice; or 8 ounces rice noodles

14 ounces firm tofu, drained

3 tablespoons canola oil, divided

kosher salt

1 sweet potato, diced

1 cup chopped red onion

1 (14-ounce) can unsweetened coconut milk

1 cup vegetable broth or water

2 tablespoons green curry paste plus additional to taste

2 tablespoons reduced sodium soy sauce or tamari (optional)

4 packed cups baby kale or spinach (about 4 ounces), washed

1 cup chopped fresh or frozen green beans

fresh cilantro, sesame seeds, and sesame oil for garnish

MAKE IT YOURSELF

Vegetable Broth (p. 293)

Cook rice (technique on p. 309). If using noodles, cook, drain, and rinse under cold water to stop the cooking process. Set aside. Press the tofu for at least 20 minutes (technique on p. 311). Cut into ½-inch cubes.

Heat 2 tablespoons oil in a large skillet and add the cubed tofu and a pinch of salt. Cook until lightly browned, about 10 minutes, stirring here and there to cook evenly. Remove from the pan and set aside.

In the same pan, heat the remaining 1 tablespoon oil. Add the diced sweet potato and red onion. Cook for 3–4 minutes, stirring occasionally.

Add the coconut milk, broth or water, green curry paste, and optional soy sauce. Simmer for 10 minutes on medium heat until the sweet potato has softened.

Add the baby kale and green beans and cook until greens are just wilted and bright green. Stir in the cooked tofu. Taste and season with additional salt and green curry paste, as desired.

Serve hot over rice or rice noodles. Garnish with cilantro, sesame seeds, and sesame oil.

SUSTAINABILITY STEPS

A motto I use often in health coaching is "progress, not perfection." We are all on a journey, and what matters is that we keep moving forward. Progress looks like one, often small, successful step at a time.

I got a running start early in life on my sustainability journey, thanks to being raised by environmentally conscious parents in an environmentally conscious state. I've had a lifetime of support and experience in making eco-friendly choices. These days my family and I grow much of our own food in our ever-expanding gardens. This year I grew grain for the first time, experimenting with amaranth for both its spinach-like greens and mature seed grain—inspiring the Ancient Grains Hot Cereal (p. 56). Harvest season is an intense but rewarding time of saucing, canning, drying, and freezing foods. My favorite thing to cook during peak garden season is Ratatouille (p. 151), and I always make sure to freeze plenty in quart containers. When a deep blanket of snow covers the garden, there is nothing better than thawing out this sun-kissed vegetable stew. It warms me, nourishing both body and soul.

I am learning more and more all the time about how to make things myself so as to decrease packaging waste that comes with most store-bought items. With a food processor, making mayonnaise, butter, tahini, nut butters, hummus, and pesto is easy, inexpensive and rewarding. Beyond food, I've had fun experimenting with recipes for homemade body care products and household cleansers. Making your own stuff is satisfying. It is a skill that builds up my self-sufficiency while deepening my understanding and appreciation for whatever it is I'm creating.

I feel empowered when I make small steps toward sustainability. When I get discouraged, I try to remember what I tell others: progress, not perfection!

Heather

Thai Veggie Brown Rice Bowl

Packed with veggie nutrients and plant-based protein, this flavorful rice or noodle bowl will be sure to satisfy.

SERVES 4

1 cup uncooked brown basmati rice; or
8 ounces rice noodles

14 ounces extra-firm tofu, drained

3 tablespoons canola oil, divided

1 head broccoli, chopped into florets

4 carrots, julienned

½ cup Peanut Sauce (p. 252)

fresh cilantro and sriracha for garnish

Cook rice (technique on p. 309). If using noodles, cook, drain, and rinse under cold water to stop the cooking process.

Press the tofu for at least 20 minutes (technique on p. 311). Cut into ½-inch cubes. Add 1 tablespoon oil to a large skillet and fry tofu, flipping occasionally, until cubes are lightly browned. Remove from skillet and set aside.

Heat the remaining 2 tablespoons oil in the skillet over medium heat and sauté the broccoli and carrots for about 5 minutes.

Assemble bowls by dividing rice, tofu, and veggies between each bowl. Dress each serving with 2 tablespoons peanut sauce drizzled over top. Garnish with cilantro and sriracha as desired.

NOTE: Save broccoli stem to use in Cruciferous Cranberry Crunch Salad (p. 76)

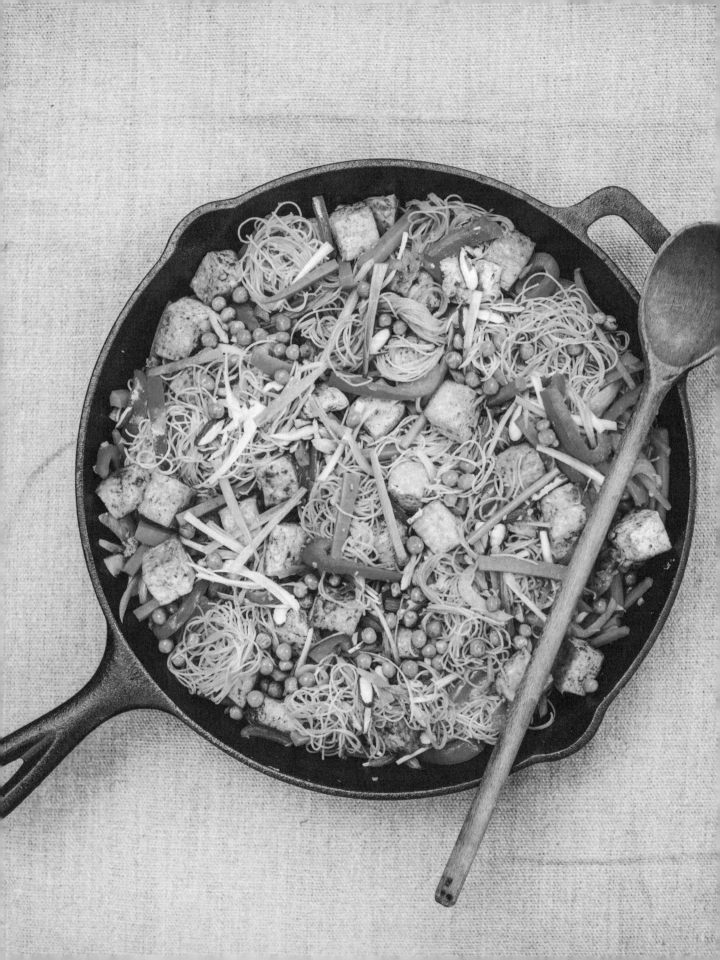

Singapore Street-Style Noodles

A favorite on southeast Asian restaurant menus, this brown rice noodle version is topped with curried almonds rather than the more traditional scrambled egg. If you are unable to find very thin rice noodles (maifun) in the Asian food section of your market, substitute vermicelli pasta.

SERVES 4

14 ounces firm or extra firm tofu

8 ounces thin maifun rice noodles (or vermicelli)

¼ cup reduced sodium soy sauce or tamari

¼ cup vegetable broth or water

1 tablespoon curry powder

1 teaspoon honey

¼ teaspoon sriracha hot sauce (optional)

¼ cup slivered or sliced almonds

¼ teaspoon ground turmeric

2 tablespoons canola oil, divided

1 onion, julienned

1 red bell pepper, julienned

2 carrots, julienned

½ cup fresh or frozen peas or snow peas

1 tablespoon minced garlic

1 tablespoon grated fresh ginger

2 green onions, julienned

4 lime wedges

MAKE IT YOURSELF

Vegetable Broth (p. 293)

Press tofu at least 20 minutes (technique on p. 311). Cut into ½-inch cubes.

Cook rice noodles. Drain and rinse under cold water to stop the cooking process. Set aside.

In a small bowl, whisk together soy sauce, broth, curry powder, honey, and optional sriracha.

Prepare all remaining ingredients. This stir-fry cooks fast, so you want everything measured and chopped before you begin to cook.

Heat a large skillet over medium heat. Add almonds and turmeric. Stir until fragrant, approximately 1 minute. Set toasted almonds aside.

Return skillet to medium heat. Add 1 tablespoon oil, cubed tofu, and 1 tablespoon of the prepared sauce. Cook for 5–10 minutes, stirring occasionally, until tofu is starting to brown on at least two sides. Remove tofu from the skillet and set aside with the noodles.

Add the remaining 1 tablespoon oil, onion, bell pepper, carrots, and peas to the skillet. Cook for about 3 minutes on high heat, stirring often. Add garlic and ginger. Cook 1 minute more.

Add noodles and remaining sauce to the stir-fried vegetables. Stir gently, mixing until sauce coats everything (a pasta fork works well for easy mixing). Remove from heat and top with tofu. Serve with toasted almonds, green onions, and a lime wedge to squeeze over the top of the noodles if desired.

Tempeh Stir-Fry with Miso Teriyaki Sauce

Fermented foods such as tempeh (soybean cake) and miso (soybean paste) contain beneficial probiotics. Combining these probiotics with prebiotics (ginger, garlic, green onions, fiber-rich vegetables) creates what is called a synbiotic stir-fry. Great for your gut, and great tasting too.

SERVES 4

---

1 cup uncooked brown rice; or 8 ounces rice noodles or lo mein noodles

STIR-FRY

8 ounces tempeh or Seitan (p. 195)

2 tablespoons canola oil, divided

4-5 cups julienned vegetables, such as carrots, bell peppers, onions, broccoli, zucchini, snap peas

3 cloves garlic, minced

1 teaspoon grated fresh ginger

1 (8-ounce) can pineapple chunks, drained (reserve juice)

SAUCE

½ cup water

¼ cup pineapple juice (reserved from can)

2 tablespoons reduced sodium soy sauce or tamari

1 tablespoon miso paste or additional soy sauce

1 tablespoon cornstarch

2 chopped green onions

¼ teaspoon hot red pepper flakes (optional)

Cook rice (technique on p. 309). If using noodles, cook, drain, and rinse under cold water to stop the cooking process.

Cut tempeh or seitan into bite-sized pieces, roughly ¼ x 1 x 1 inch.

Prepare vegetables for stir-fry. Cutting into thin strips (julienne cut) works well. Uniform sizes are important so that the vegetables cook evenly.

Whisk together all sauce ingredients in a small bowl until well combined.

Heat 1 tablespoon oil in a large skillet over medium-high heat. Add tempeh and cook until golden brown, stirring occasionally. Remove tempeh from skillet and set aside.

Add julienned vegetables to the hot skillet with the remaining 1 tablespoon oil. Stir-fry until tender but still crisp, 3–5 minutes. Add garlic and ginger and cook for 1 minute.

Add pineapple, tempeh, and sauce. Stir until everything is coated and sauce begins to thicken, about 1 minute (a pasta fork works well for easy mixing).

Serve over your choice of cooked rice or noodles, or enjoy it on its own.

Quinoa Enchilada Skillet

This single-skillet meal makes cooking and cleanup easy. Serve as is, use as a filling inside a soft tortilla, or use for stuffed peppers. Makes great leftovers!

SERVES 4

1 tablespoon olive oil

2 cloves garlic, minced

1 jalapeño pepper, minced (remove seeds if you prefer less heat)

6 green onions, thinly sliced (both white and green parts)

2 cups diced zucchini

1 cup fresh or frozen corn kernels

1 cup uncooked quinoa

1½ cups cooked black beans (reserve cooking liquid/aquafaba)

1 cup liquid (reserved aquafaba, broth, or water)

3 cups Enchilada Sauce (p. 245); or 1 (28-ounce) can fire-roasted diced tomatoes

1 teaspoon chili powder

1 teaspoon ground cumin

¼ teaspoon kosher salt

¼ teaspoon freshly ground black pepper

2 tablespoons chopped fresh cilantro

juice of ½ lime

1 avocado, diced

shredded cheese, such as cheddar or Monterey Jack (optional)

hot sauce (optional)

In a large skillet with a lid (so that it can be covered later), heat oil over medium-high heat. Add garlic, jalapeño, and white part of green onions (reserve green part). Stir and cook until fragrant, about 1 minute.

Add zucchini, corn, quinoa, black beans, 1 cup liquid, enchilada sauce, chili powder, cumin, salt, and pepper. Bring to a boil, then reduce heat, cover, and simmer on low for 20 minutes. Remove from heat.

Stir in green part of green onions, cilantro, and lime juice. Top with avocado, optional cheese, and hot sauce, if desired.

Stuffed pepper variation: Cut 6 large bell peppers in half vertically. Remove and compost seeds and stems. Rub pepper halves with oil. Place in a lightly oiled 9 x 13-inch baking pan. Stuff pepper halves with quinoa mixture. Cover pan with aluminum foil. Place in a cold oven and turn heat to 400°F. Start timing and bake 30 minutes. Remove foil. Top with shredded cheese, if desired. Bake another 15 minutes until peppers are soft and starting to brown.

MAKE IT YOURSELF

Canned Diced Tomatoes (p. 274)

Cauliflower Tacos

You can really get some heat with these tacos or keep the spice level mild; just adjust the adobo sauce to your taste. If you opt to make our refried beans and tortillas with this recipe, we encourage you to make them in advance or else give yourself about 2 hours from start to finish.

SERVES 6–8

TACOS

1 small head cauliflower, cut into small florets and stem thinly sliced into bite-sized pieces

2 individual chipotle peppers in adobo sauce, chopped (about 2 tablespoons)

1 tablespoon adobo sauce (from chipotles)

1½ tablespoons olive oil

kosher salt and freshly ground black pepper

1¼ cups Refried Beans, black bean variation (p. 198)

4 cups Cilantro Lime Slaw (p. 201)

8 whole wheat tortillas

fresh cilantro for garnish

CHIPOTLE MAYO

½ cup mayonnaise

½ tablespoon adobo sauce (from chipotles)

1 clove garlic, minced

1 teaspoon freshly squeezed lime juice plus additional to taste

1 teaspoon honey (optional)

kosher salt and freshly ground black pepper

Combine cauliflower, chopped chipotle peppers, adobo sauce, oil, and a pinch of salt and pepper. Mix to combine. Transfer to a baking sheet and spread out in a single layer. Place in a cold oven and turn to 400°F. Start timing and bake for 25 minutes.

While cauliflower is roasting, make the chipotle mayo: In a small bowl, combine mayonnaise, adobo sauce, garlic, lime juice, optional honey, and a pinch of salt. Whisk until smooth. Taste and adjust the seasoning, adding more salt, pepper, and lime juice as desired.

To assemble the tacos: For each tortilla, layer a scant ¼ cup refried beans, ½ cup roasted cauliflower, ½ cup slaw, and drizzle with 1 tablespoon chipotle mayo. Garnish with cilantro if desired.

MAKE IT YOURSELF

Mayonnaise (p. 285)

Chipotle Peppers in Adobo Sauce (p. 279)

Whole Wheat Tortillas (p. 286)

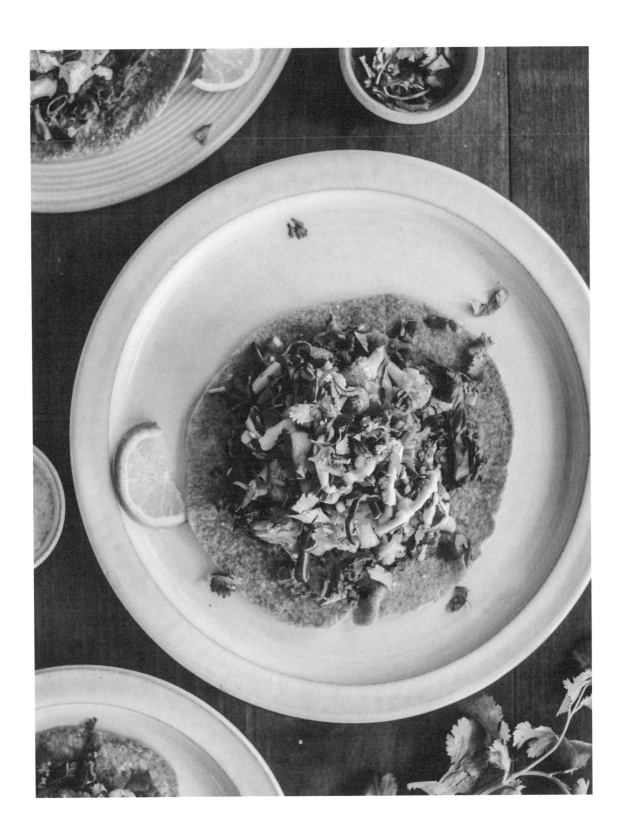

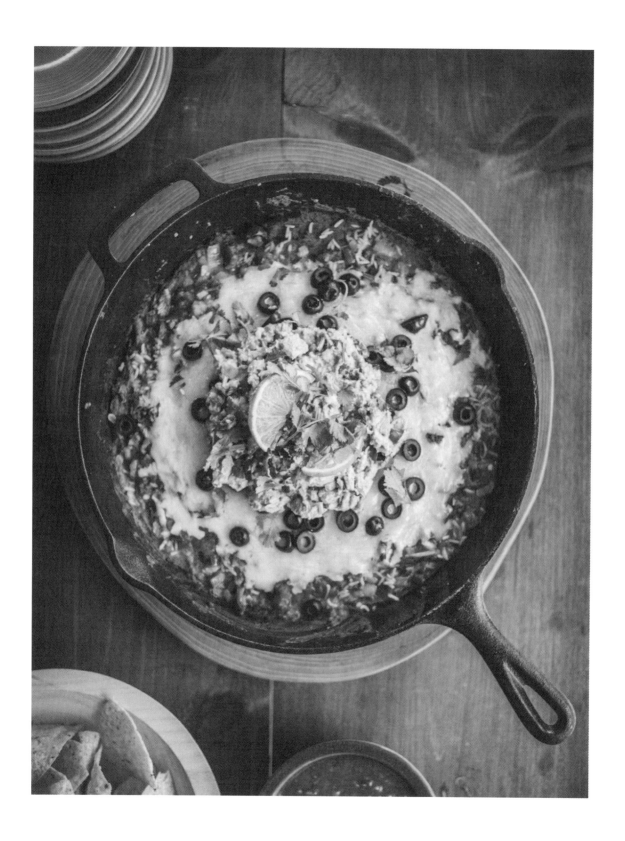

Seven-Layer Burrito Pan

Use this as a filling for burritos or simply dip your chip right in for a nacho night. Prep everything ahead in the layered dish and it'll be ready to bake whenever you are ready to eat.

SERVES 6

½ cup uncooked brown rice

1 tablespoon canola oil

1 green bell pepper, chopped

1 onion, chopped

2½ cups Refried Beans (p. 198)

1 cup Fresh Salsa (p. 254)

1 cup (4 ounces) shredded cheddar cheese

½ cup sliced black olives

2 avocados, sliced; or 1 cup Guacamole (p. 257)

fresh cilantro for garnish

MAKE IT YOURSELF

Whole Wheat Tortillas (p. 286)

Cook rice (technique on p. 309). Set aside.

In an oven-safe skillet (such as cast iron or all stainless steel) over medium heat, add oil, pepper, and onion. Sauté until softened and beginning to brown, about 5 minutes. Remove from skillet and set aside.

Layer ingredients in skillet. Start with refried beans as a base, followed by the sautéed pepper and onion, then cooked rice, salsa, cheddar cheese, and olives.

Place in a cold oven and turn to 350°F. Start timing and bake for 20 minutes until warmed through.

Top with avocado or guacamole and garnish with cilantro if desired.

Serve as a dip with tortilla chips, or spoon into soft tortillas to make burrito wraps.

Frozen burrito variation: For healthy and homemade fast food, make your own frozen burritos. Scoop some burrito mixture, minus the avocado, into whole wheat tortillas. Wrap up and freeze. To cook, microwave a frozen burrito for 2–3 minutes total: 60–90 seconds one side, then flip and cook 60–90 seconds on the other side. Let sit for 1 minute before eating.

Chorizo Quesadillas

These quesadillas are a great way to use up any extra of our Spicy Cauliflower Walnut Chorizo. Any leftover sautéed or roasted veggies you have hanging around the fridge could be added in too.

SERVES 4

8 whole wheat tortillas

1 cup (4 ounces) shredded Monterey Jack or cheddar cheese or a combination

2 cups Spicy Cauliflower Walnut Chorizo (p. 197)

1½ cups Fresh Salsa (p. 254)

1 cup Guacamole (p. 257)

chopped fresh cilantro and lime wedges for garnish

Build quesadillas by placing a tortilla in a skillet and layering with 2 tablespoons cheese, ½ cup chorizo, another 2 tablespoons cheese, and another tortilla. Cook over medium-high heat for 3–5 minutes, flip, and cook an additional 3 minutes.

Serve with fresh salsa and guacamole on the side. Garnish with chopped cilantro and lime wedges, if desired.

MAKE IT YOURSELF

Whole Wheat Tortillas (p. 286)

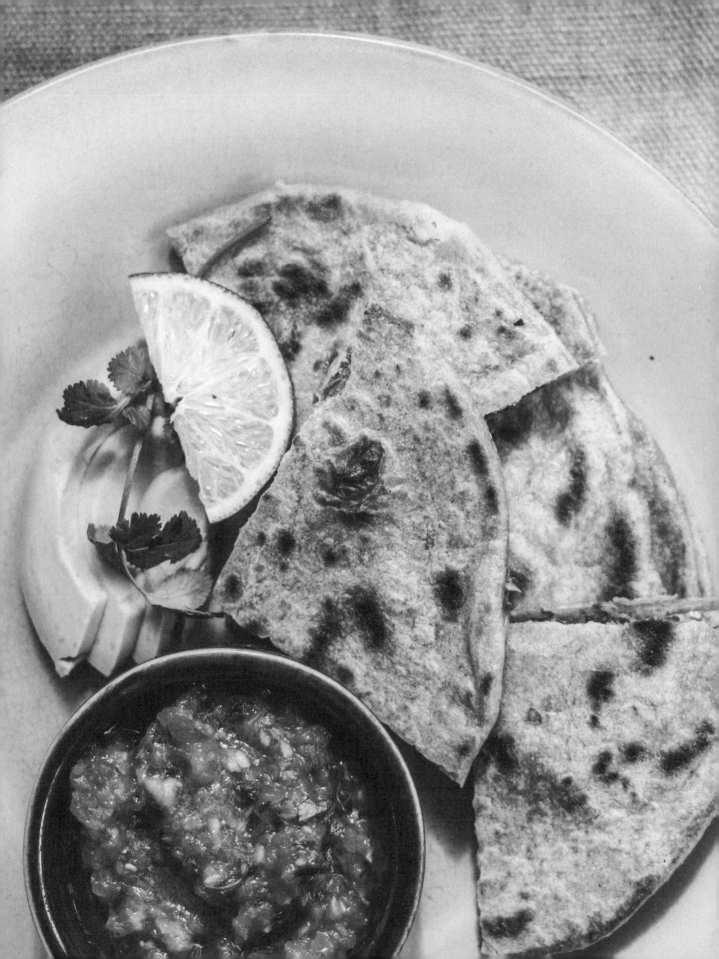

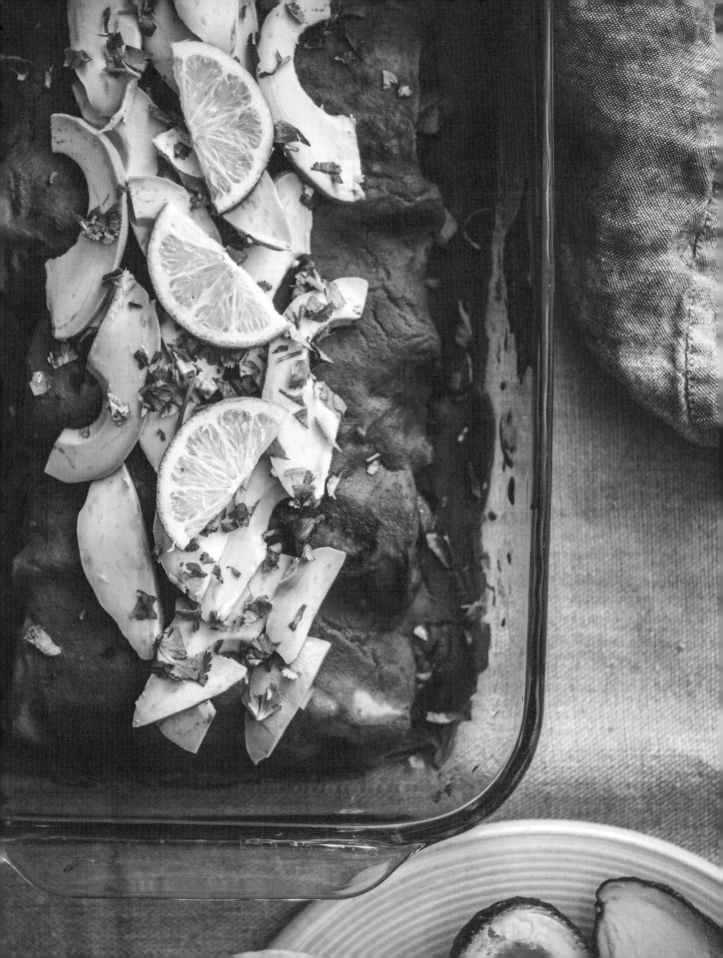

Sweet Potato and Black Bean Enchiladas

These vegan enchiladas are so full of flavor that you won't even miss the cheese, but cheese can be added.

SERVES 6

6 whole wheat tortillas

2 cups finely diced sweet potatoes

1 tablespoon olive oil

1 onion, chopped

2 cloves garlic, minced

1 teaspoon chili powder, or to taste

½ teaspoon ground cumin

¾ teaspoon kosher salt

¼ teaspoon freshly ground black pepper

1 green bell pepper, chopped

2 ounces spinach, chopped (about 2 packed cups)

1½ cups cooked black beans

3 cups Enchilada Sauce (p. 245), divided

juice of ½ lime

6 ounces cheddar cheese, shredded (optional)

fresh cilantro, sliced avocado, and thinly sliced green onions for garnish

MAKE IT YOURSELF

Whole Wheat Tortillas (p. 286)

Lightly oil a 9 x 13-inch baking pan.

Place the sweet potatoes in a medium saucepan and add enough water to cover. Bring the water to a boil, then reduce the heat to medium-high and simmer for 5–7 minutes, or until sweet potatoes are fork tender. Drain and set aside.

In a large skillet, heat the oil over medium heat. Add the onion and sauté for about 5 minutes until translucent. Stir in garlic, chili powder, cumin, salt, and pepper. Cook until fragrant, about 30 seconds.

Add the cooked sweet potatoes, bell pepper, spinach, and beans and cook for a few minutes more, or until the spinach is wilted.

Remove the skillet from the heat and stir in ¼ cup enchilada sauce and lime juice.

Spread 1 cup enchilada sauce on the bottom of the prepared pan. Scoop ¾ cup sweet potato filling onto each tortilla. Roll up the tortillas and place them seam side down in the pan. Spread the remaining enchilada sauce over the tortillas. If you have leftover filling, either add it to the pan on one side or save to eat later.

Place enchiladas in a cold oven and turn to 350°F. Start timing and bake, uncovered, for 25 minutes.

Garnish with cilantro, avocado, and green onions if desired.

Three Sisters Succotash Enchiladas

Corn, beans, and squash, known as the Three Sisters, cook together into a simple succotash, which is then used to stuff these enchiladas (but also makes a great side dish). We give you the option to make everything from scratch. If you can make the tortillas, sauce, and succotash ahead of time, the enchiladas come together quickly. A very satisfying main-dish meal that is well worth the work.

SERVES 8

SUCCOTASH

3 cups chopped fresh or frozen green beans; or 1½ cups cooked black beans (reserve cooking liquid/aquafaba)

1 tablespoon canola oil

3 cups diced summer squash (such as zucchini, yellow squash, or patty pan)

2 cups fresh or frozen corn

2–4 tablespoons liquid (reserved aquafaba, broth, or water)

¼ teaspoon kosher salt

⅛ teaspoon freshly ground black pepper

ENCHILADAS

3 cups Enchilada Sauce (p. 245), divided

8 whole wheat tortillas

2 cups (8 ounces) shredded cheddar cheese, divided

chopped fresh cilantro and diced avocado for garnish

MAKE IT YOURSELF

Whole Wheat Tortillas (p. 286)

Prepare the succotash: In a saucepan, add green beans and enough water to cover them (if using cooked black beans, skip this step). Bring saucepan to a boil over medium-high heat. Cover and simmer until beans are tender. Times will vary: for thin French green beans (haricots verts), simmer about 10 minutes; for bigger green beans, it may take up to 20 minutes.

Heat oil in a large skillet. Sauté the summer squash and corn for about 5 minutes. Stir occasionally. Add cooked beans and 2 tablespoons liquid. Cook for another 5 minutes, stirring occasionally. Add more liquid as needed to prevent the skillet from going dry. Add salt and pepper.

Assemble enchiladas: Oil a 9 x 13-inch baking pan. Spread 1 cup enchilada sauce on the bottom of the pan. Down the center of each tortilla, put ½ cup succotash and 2 tablespoons cheddar cheese. Roll up each tortilla and place seam side down in the pan. Spread the remaining 2 cups enchilada sauce over top. Cover pan with a lid or aluminum foil. Place in a cold oven and turn to 350°F. Start timing and bake for 30 minutes. Remove cover and sprinkle on the remaining 1 cup cheese. Continue baking, uncovered, until cheese is melted, about 10 minutes. Garnish with cilantro and avocado, if desired.

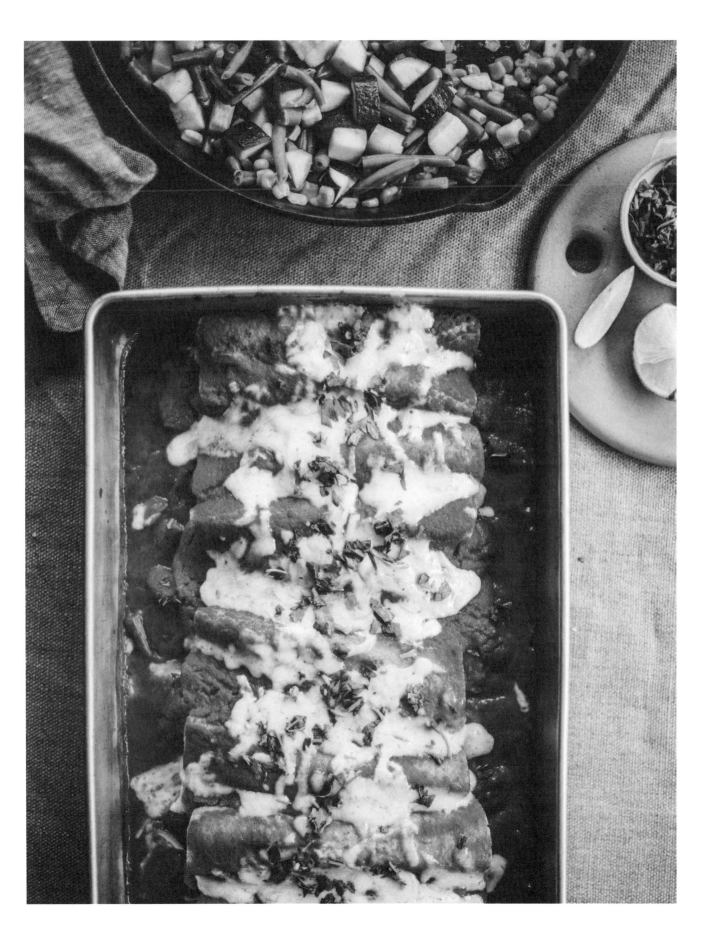

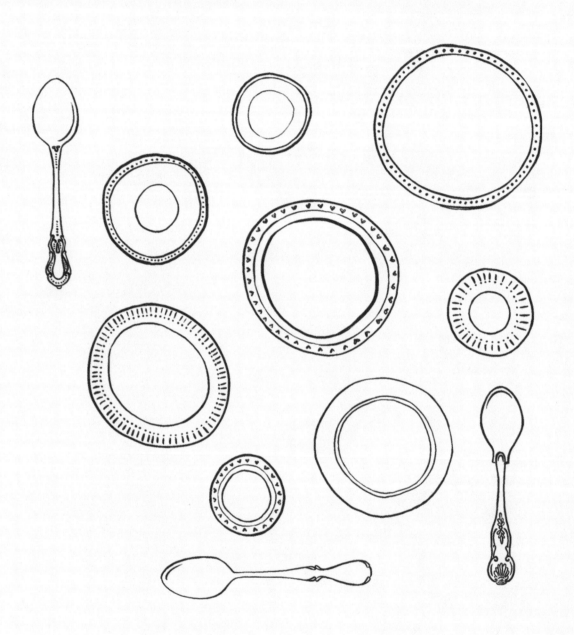

Sides and
Supports

———

Beet Green Sauté

Too often discarded, beet greens are rich in nutrients and make for a quick side dish not unlike Swiss chard. Next time you prepare beets for a recipe (such as our Roasted Beet Salad, p. 70), save the greens so all edible portions of the plant are used. Adjust the recipe to accommodate the amount of beet greens you have on hand. Substitute other greens such as dandelion, collards, Swiss chard, or spinach.

SERVES 4

1 pound beet greens (stems and leaves from about 6 medium beets)

1 tablespoon olive oil

2 cloves garlic, minced

¼ teaspoon kosher salt

¼ teaspoon hot red pepper flakes

⅛ teaspoon freshly ground black pepper

2 teaspoons freshly squeezed lemon juice or vinegar

Wash beet greens. Separate stems and leaves. Chop stems into 1-inch pieces. Roughly chop leaves.

Place beet stems in a medium saucepan. Cover with water and bring to a boil. Cook for about 5 minutes. Add the chopped leaves. Stir until wilted. Remove from heat and let greens sit in the hot water.

Heat oil in a skillet over medium heat. Add garlic, salt, hot red pepper flakes, and black pepper. Cook until garlic is fragrant, no more than 1 minute.

Using a slotted spoon, remove beet stems and leaves from the saucepan and add them directly to the skillet. Sauté for about 5 minutes, or until all the liquid has cooked off. Turn off heat. Stir in lemon juice.

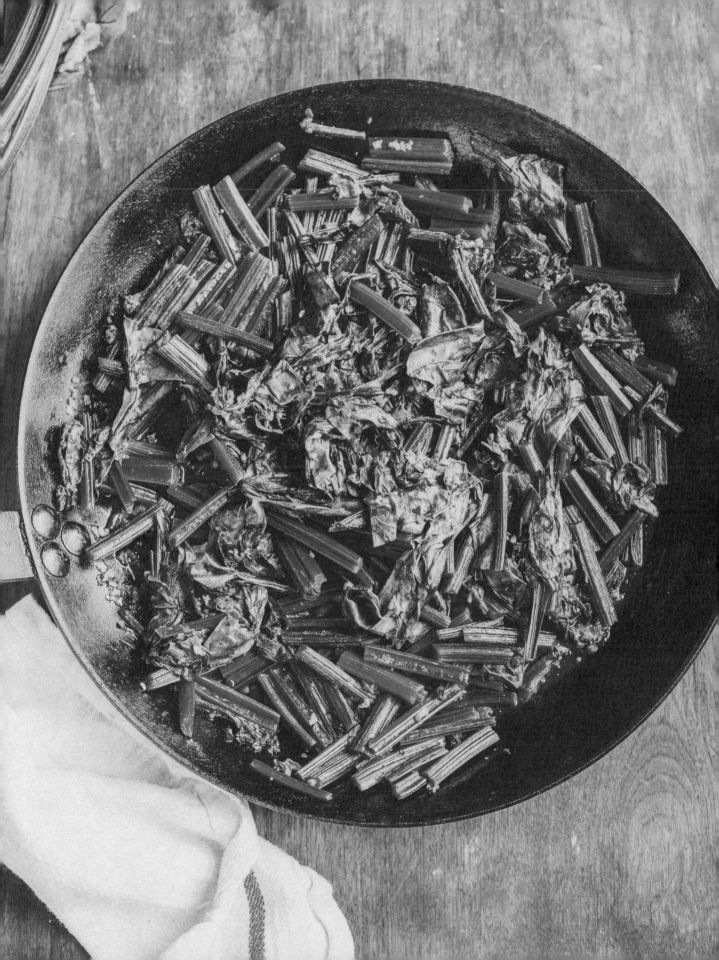

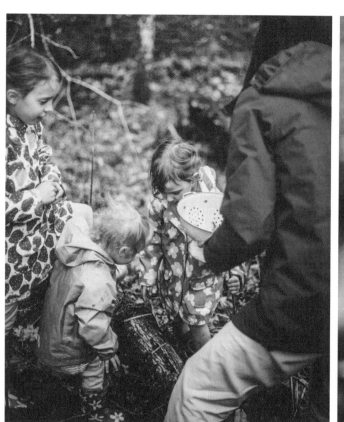
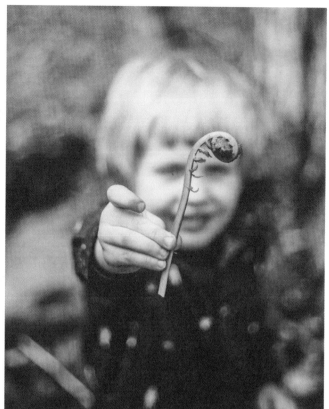
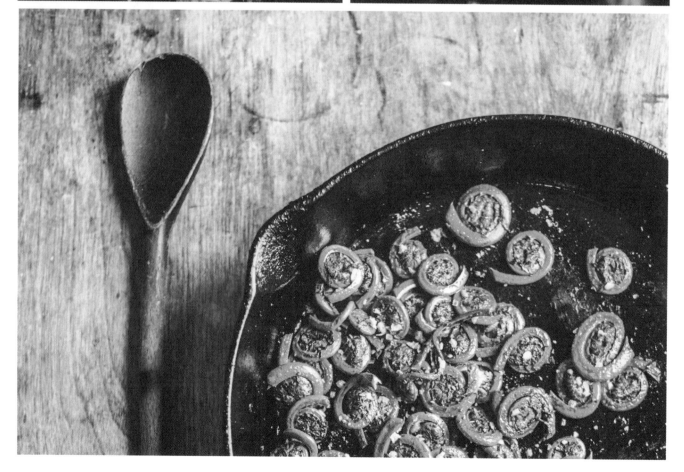

Foraged Fiddleheads

Nothing says spring or local, in-season eating like this simple sautéed side dish. Fiddleheads—the young fronds of an ostrich fern prior to unfurling—can be gathered from the awakening landscape. Never pick more than half the fiddleheads emerging from a clump, called a crown. In their coiled form, they do indeed look like the head of a fiddle. You could substitute ramps, another ethereal wildcrafted spring green, in place of the garlic.

SERVES: 6

1 pound fiddleheads (about 5 cups)

salt and freshly ground black pepper

1 tablespoon olive oil

1 tablespoon butter

4 cloves garlic, minced; or 4-6 ramps, finely chopped

Wash fiddleheads in bowl of cold water, swishing them around to rinse away the brown papery husks. You may need to do this water bath several times until clean. Trim ends if needed.

Bring a pot of water to boil. Add a pinch of salt if desired. Boil fiddleheads for 10 minutes. (The cooking water likely will have turned brown; this is to be expected.) Drain. Rinse cooked fiddleheads under cold water or plunge into an ice bath to stop the cooking process. Set aside.

In a skillet, heat oil and butter over medium heat. Add garlic. Sauté for 30 seconds (if using ramps, sauté for 2 minutes). Add drained fiddleheads and continue to sauté for another 3 minutes. Season with salt and pepper to taste.

Serving suggestion: Eat fiddleheads on their own or try mixing together with Sautéed Mushrooms Marinated in Garlic (p. 204). These two sides complement each other.

MAKE IT YOURSELF

Butter (p. 282)

Spinach and White Bean Sauté

There are many different white beans, and just about any will do for this recipe. The most common white beans found in stores are navy beans, cannellini beans, and Great Northern beans. While there are slight size differences, their flavor profiles are similar enough that they can be used interchangeably.

SERVES 4

2 tablespoons olive oil

3 cloves garlic, minced

⅛–¼ teaspoon hot red pepper flakes

10 ounces spinach (baby, chopped mature leaves, or thawed from frozen and drained)

1½ cups cooked white beans (reserve cooking liquid/aquafaba)

¼–½ cup liquid (reserved aquafaba, broth, or water)

1 teaspoon freshly squeezed lemon juice

⅛ teaspoon kosher salt

⅛ teaspoon freshly ground black pepper

extra-virgin olive oil for drizzling

Heat oil in a medium saucepan or skillet over medium heat. Sauté garlic, hot red pepper flakes, and spinach until the spinach is warm and wilted. You may need to add the spinach several handfuls at a time, then allow it to wilt down and add more until all has been incorporated. Stir in beans and ¼ cup liquid. Cook until heated through. Add more liquid if needed to prevent skillet from going dry. Remove from heat. Stir in lemon juice, salt, and pepper, adjusting to taste. Drizzle with a little extra-virgin olive oil just before serving.

Slow Cooker Maple "Baked" Beans

A vegetarian alternative to traditional baked beans, which are usually cooked with salt pork or bacon. We use soy sauce to achieve the salty, umami taste. A dark-colored, robust-tasting maple syrup is preferred. This is a slow cooker recipe. If you have a multicooker, you can take advantage of three features: pressure-cook, sauté/brown, and slow-cook.

SERVES 10

1 pound dry white beans such as navy or soldier beans (about 2 ½ cups; reserve cooking liquid/aquafaba)

1½ cups liquid (reserved aquafaba, broth, or water)

½ cup maple syrup

¼ cup tomato paste

1 tablespoon reduced sodium soy sauce or tamari

1 teaspoon dry mustard

1 teaspoon kosher salt

1 tablespoon canola oil

1 onion, finely diced

Soak and cook dry beans (technique on p. 313).

Whisk together 1½ cups liquid, maple syrup, tomato paste, soy sauce, dry mustard, and salt.

Heat oil in a small skillet over medium heat. Add onion and cook for 5 minutes, stirring occasionally.

In the pot of your slow cooker, combine sautéed onion, beans, and liquid mixture. Cover and cook on low for 8 hours. The sauce will thicken as it cools.

Baked variation: Follow directions above but instead of putting everything into your slow cooker, combine everything in a covered 2½ quart casserole dish. Cover and cook at 250°F for 4-5 hours, until beans are very tender. Remove cover. Bake an additional 45 minutes, or until top is crusty.

Maple Paprika Roasted Brussels Sprouts

The combination of sweet and spice is oh so nice. Crispy brussels sprouts leaves just might remind you of barbecue-flavored chips.

SERVES 6

---

1 pound brussels sprouts, trimmed and halved (quartered if large)

2 tablespoons olive oil

1 tablespoon maple syrup

¾ teaspoon paprika or smoked paprika

½ teaspoon kosher salt

¼ teaspoon freshly ground black pepper

Lightly oil a baking sheet. (Alternatively, line with eco-friendly parchment paper for easy cleanup.) Toss all ingredients together in a large bowl, mixing well to coat. Spread out the brussels sprouts in a single layer on the baking sheet. Place in a cold oven and turn to 450°F. Start timing and roast for 25 minutes. If even browning is desired, stir about halfway through the cooking time.

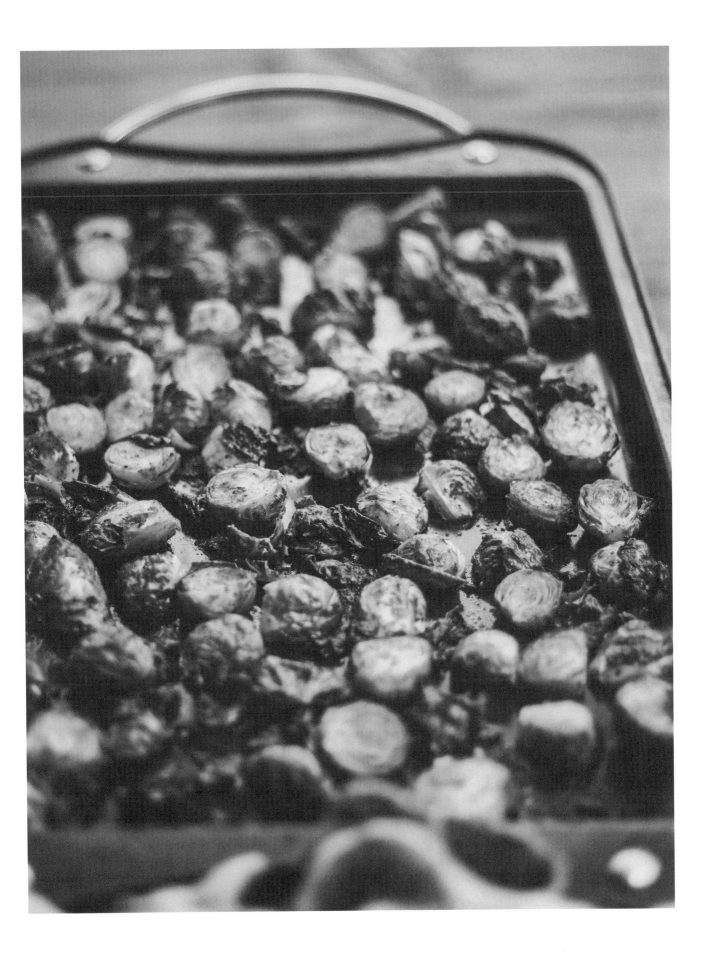

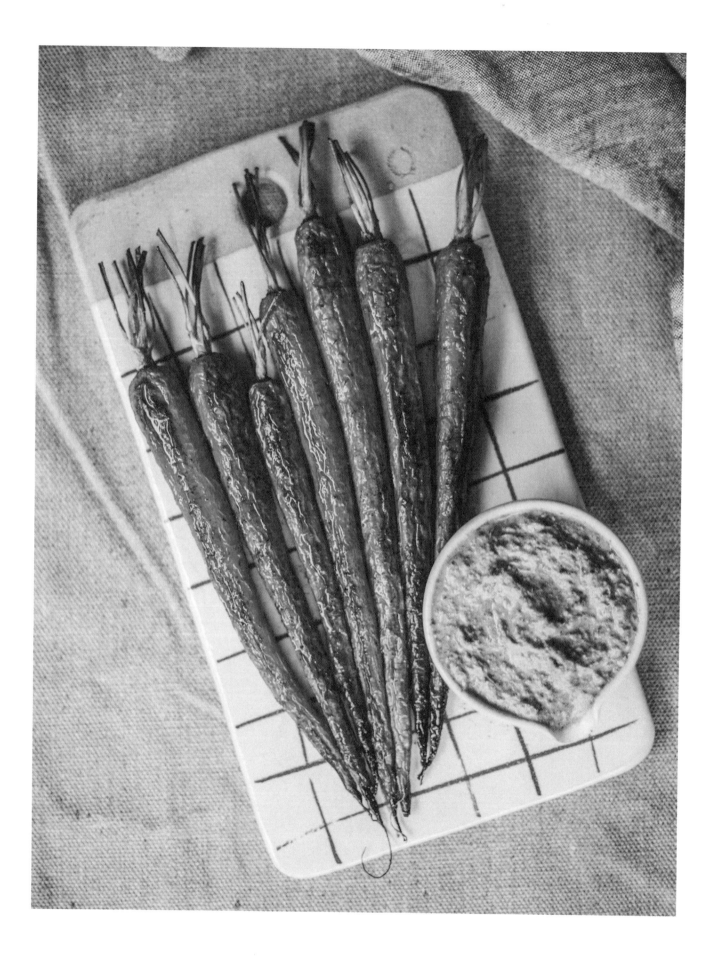

Spice-Rubbed Roasted Carrots

Roasting brings out natural sweetness in the carrots to complement the spices you've rubbed on their surface. Serve as a stand-alone side or with Carrot Top Pesto (p. 248).

SERVES 6

1 pound carrots

1 tablespoon olive oil

¼ teaspoon ground coriander

¼ teaspoon ground cumin

¼ teaspoon paprika

Cut thick carrots into large spears, or leave whole if they are on the thin side. In a large bowl, combine carrots, oil, coriander, cumin, and paprika. Use your hands or a mixing spoon to rub the spices onto the carrots.

Spread out spiced carrots on a baking sheet in a single layer. Place in a cold oven and turn to 450°F. Start timing and roast in the oven for about 30 minutes, or until carrots are tender. Cook time will largely depend on how big your carrots are. If even browning is desired, stir about halfway through the cooking time.

Roasted Veggies for All Seasons

Roasting brings out the best in vegetables, no matter the time of year. The high heat and extended cooking time caramelizes the veggies, transforming them into something irresistible. Flavor vegetables with herbs and spices that suit the season.

SERVES 6

---

6 cups diced seasonal vegetables (see instructions)

SPRING MEDLEY WITH PESTO

2 tablespoons olive oil

½ teaspoon kosher salt

Classic Basil Pesto (p. 247) as desired

freshly grated Parmesan cheese

SIMPLY SALTED SUMMER MIX

2 cloves garlic, chopped

2 tablespoons olive oil

½ teaspoon kosher salt

freshly ground black pepper

CURRIED FALL VEGETABLES

2 tablespoons curry powder

2 tablespoons olive oil

1 tablespoon minced fresh ginger; or 1 teaspoon ground

½ teaspoon kosher salt

HONEY ROASTED WINTER ROOTS

¼ cup honey

2 tablespoons olive oil

½ teaspoon kosher salt

Prepare your seasonal selection of vegetables: Spring options include asparagus, parsnips, radishes, and shallots. Summer options include broccoli, bell peppers, summer squash, and zucchini. Fall options include cauliflower, eggplant, potato, and onion. Winter options include carrot, sweet potato, white potato, beets, turnip, and winter squash. Dice the vegetables into uniform pieces, as similar sizes will cook evenly. A large ¾- to 1-inch dice is recommended.

In a large bowl, mix the diced vegetables with the ingredients listed under your selected version (except for the spring version; the pesto and Parmesan cheese should be mixed in after roasting). Stir until well combined.

Spread vegetables onto two baking sheets in a single layer. Place in a cold oven and turn to 450°F. Start timing and roast for 30–40 minutes until tender and caramelized. Roasting time will depend on the thickness and variety of the veggies. If even browning is desired, stir about halfway through the cooking time. Vegetables are done when tender and browned.

If making the spring medley, mix in the pesto and Parmesan cheese after roasting.

LEARNING HOW TO COOK

I learned to cook from the Internet. Pinterest became my go-to resource for cooking because I loved that I could look up food by the ingredients I had on hand while also getting good food photography. I liked that I could save a recipe while on the bus or in between classes and then easily pull it up later when making the grocery list. Yet I started noticing that using this great tool left me overwhelmed. I could make the "best tacos ever" with "life-changing guacamole"—or maybe "the most amazing oven-roasted corn"? Five-star cuisine seemed always possible, even though that guacamole was often mediocre. Even so, there was a lot I took from that experience. I eventually noticed which sources were the best and I started to go directly to specific food blogs and cooking websites that I could trust. The not-so-good recipes taught me what not to do. The more I cooked, the more confident I became in trying my own recipes and substituting something I had on hand when a certain ingredient was missing from my kitchen. Eventually I was winging entire meals. It was often confusing and overwhelming, but the takeaway was well worth it.

Jaymie

Delicata Squash Smiles

Garnishing with seasonal herbs and fruit turns this into a festive side dish for holiday meals. Use sage and cranberries at Thanksgiving or mint and pomegranate seeds at Christmas. Delicata squash have thin, tender skin and don't need to be peeled.

SERVES 6

---

3 delicata squash (about 2½ pounds); or 1 acorn squash

1 tablespoon olive oil

1 tablespoon honey (optional)

¼ teaspoon kosher salt

⅛ teaspoon freshly ground black pepper

2 tablespoons minced fresh sage or mint (optional)

¼ cup dried cranberries or fresh pomegranate seeds (optional)

Cut squash in half lengthwise, removing seeds and inner strings. If you want to roast the squash seeds for a snack (see p. 210), prep them now so they can go in the oven with the squash but on a separate baking sheet.

Slice squash into semicircles, about ¾ inch thick, to get your "smiles." Toss squash, oil, optional honey, salt, and pepper together in a large bowl, mixing well to coat. Spread the squash out in a single layer on a lightly oiled baking sheet. (Alternatively, line with eco-friendly parchment paper for easy cleanup.)

Place in a cold oven and turn to 450°F. Start timing and roast squash for 25 minutes. If even browning is desired, stir to flip squash over about halfway through the cooking time.

If desired, garnish the roasted squash with an herb (sage or mint) and fruit (dried cranberries or pomegranate seeds) at serving time.

Seitan

The "meat of wheat," seitan is high in protein and is dense and chewy, making it an excellent plant-based substitute for meat in many recipes. It has a neutral taste and will absorb flavors well of any recipe you use it in. The added nutritional yeast provides important vitamin B12, which can be hard to get in a vegan diet, as B12 is almost exclusively found in animal foods.

MAKES 1 POUND

---

1 cup vital wheat gluten

½ cup chickpea flour

½ cup nutritional yeast

2 teaspoons garlic powder

5¾ cups vegetable broth, divided

2 tablespoons reduced sodium soy sauce or tamari

1 garlic clove, halved

½ onion, sliced

MAKE IT YOURSELF

Vegetable Broth (p. 293)

USE IN THESE RECIPES

Seitan Piccata (p. 128)
Crispy Tofu Parmesan (p. 132)
Tempeh Stir-Fry (p. 168)

Mix together wheat gluten, chickpea flour, nutritional yeast, garlic powder, and ¾ cup broth until it forms a dough. Knead for several minutes until the dough becomes elastic. Shape into a disc that is about a 6-inch diameter and ¾-inch thickness. Cut disc into quarters so you have four smaller chunks.

Add seitan to a large saucepan with the remaining 5 cups broth, soy sauce, garlic clove, and onion. Seitan dough should be covered by liquid. If not, add water until covered. Seitan expands during cooking. Bring to a boil over medium heat. Cover, reduce heat, and simmer for 45 minutes. Turn off heat and allow seitan to rest in the broth for an additional 15 minutes. Remove with a slotted spoon. Once cooled, seitan can be stored in the refrigerator for up to 1 week or in the freezer for at least 1 month.

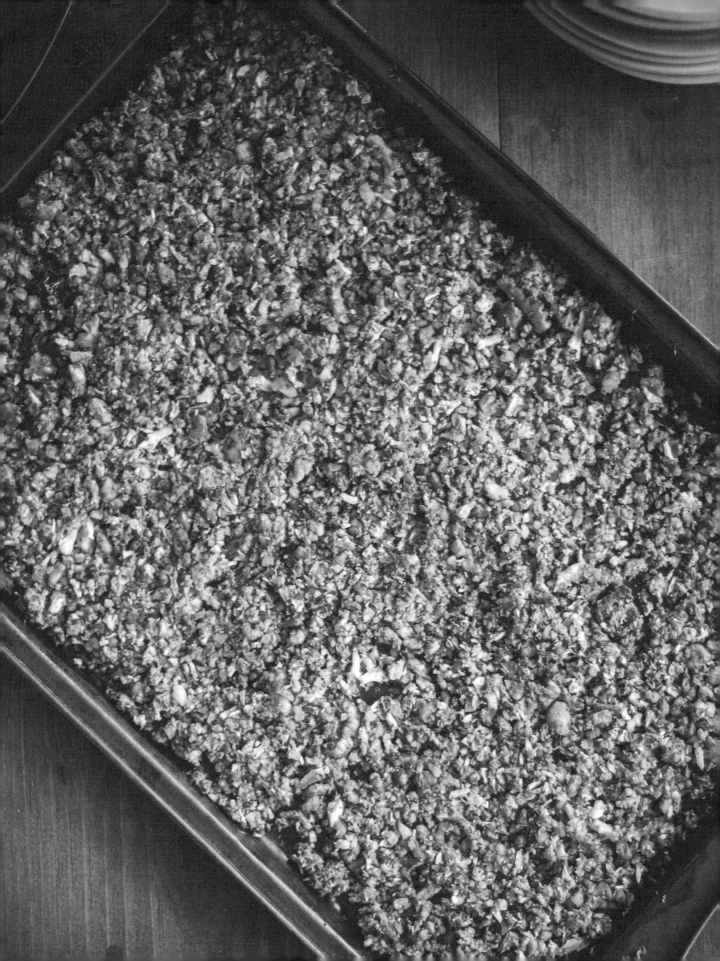

Spicy Cauliflower Walnut Chorizo

A versatile and vitamin-packed vegan alternative to chorizo, a type of pork sausage. Makes a great side for a savory breakfast meal, or use it in an entrée such as tacos, quesadillas, or a rice bowl.

MAKES 4 CUPS

1 head cauliflower, roughly chopped (both florets and stem)

2 cups walnuts

2 individual chipotle peppers in adobo sauce (p. 279)

1 tablespoon chili powder

1 teaspoon ground cumin

1 teaspoon kosher salt

¼ teaspoon garlic powder

¼ teaspoon onion powder

Lightly oil a baking sheet.

Add all ingredients into to a food processor or blender and pulse until evenly mixed and the cauliflower and walnuts are in small pieces but not pureed. (If using a blender, you may need to add 1 cup of the mixture at a time and transfer each batch to the prepared baking sheet to ensure even texture and prevent overprocessing.) Flatten the mixture onto the baking sheet until evenly distributed. Place in cold oven and turn to 350°F. Start timing and bake for 35 minutes. If even browning is desired, stir about halfway through the cooking time.

USE IN THESE RECIPES

Breakfast Tacos (p. 46)

Cauliflower Tacos (p. 170)

Chorizo Quesadillas (p. 174)

MAKE IT YOURSELF

Chipotle Peppers in Adobo Sauce (p. 279)

Refried Beans

Making your own refried beans allows you to spice them just how you like. You choose pinto or black beans and whether to start this recipe from canned or dry beans. If you have time, starting from bulk dry beans will save money and packaging waste.

MAKES 2½ CUPS

1 tablespoon canola oil

½ onion, minced

1 jalapeño pepper, minced (optional)

2 cloves garlic, minced

1 teaspoon chili powder

1 teaspoon ground cumin

¼ teaspoon kosher salt

3 cups cooked pinto or black beans (reserve cooking liquid/aquafaba)

2-4 tablespoons liquid (reserved aquafaba or freshly squeezed lime juice)

Heat oil in a large skillet over medium heat. Add onion and optional jalapeño (remove seeds if you want less heat). Cook until soft but not browned, about 3 minutes. Stir in garlic, chili powder, cumin, and salt. Cook about 1 minute to bloom the spices. Add the beans and cook until warm, about 5 minutes. Remove from heat.

Add 2 tablespoons liquid. For a chunky texture, mash with a potato masher or the back of a wooden spoon. For a creamier texture, use a food processor or blender. Add additional liquid as needed to achieve your desired consistency. Adjust seasonings to taste.

USE IN THESE RECIPES

Cauliflower Tacos (p. 170)
Seven-Layer Burrito Pan (p. 173)

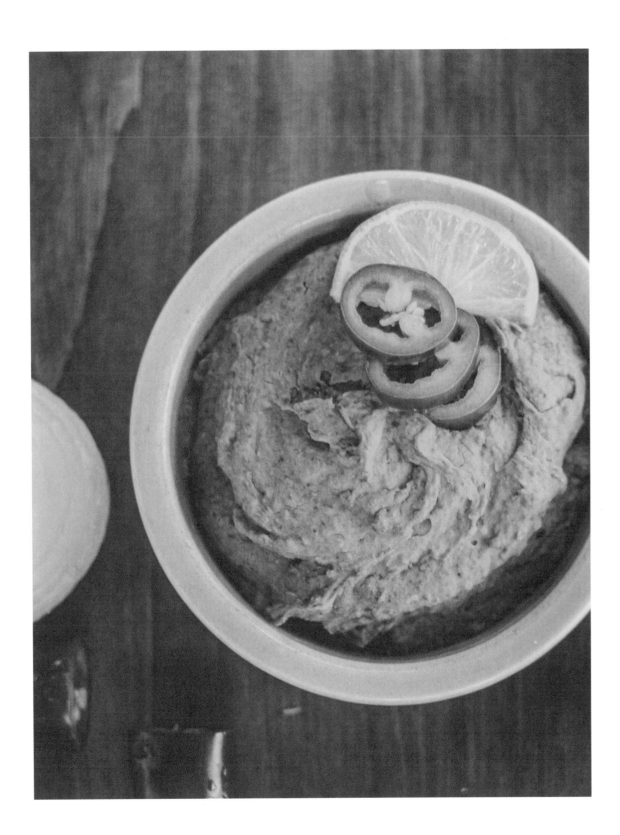

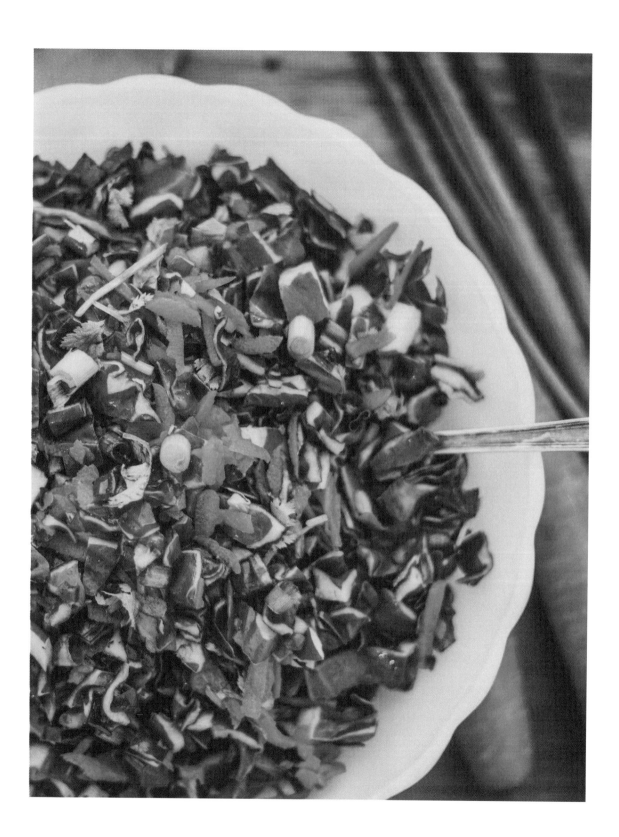

Cilantro Lime Slaw

A refreshing summertime alternative to a mayonnaise-based coleslaw. We use this slaw in tacos and wraps, but it can also stand alone as a side.

MAKES 5 CUPS

4 cups shredded red or green cabbage (approximately ½ head cabbage)

1 carrot, shredded

3 green onions, thinly sliced (both green and white parts)

2 tablespoons chopped fresh cilantro

2 tablespoons unseasoned rice vinegar

1 tablespoon canola oil

juice of ½ lime

½ teaspoon kosher salt

¼ teaspoon freshly ground black pepper

1 tablespoon honey (optional)

Combine cabbage, carrot, green onions, and cilantro.

Whisk together vinegar, oil, lime juice, salt, pepper, and optional honey.

Add dressing to the cabbage mixture and stir well to coat evenly. Adjust seasonings as desired.

USE IN THESE RECIPES

Thai Veggie Tofu Wrap (p. 117)
Cauliflower Tacos (p. 170)

Caramelized Onions

Caramelizing onions takes time, but the transformation from strong to sweet is worth the wait. A delicious addition to so many dishes, including burgers, pizza, pasta, and sandwiches.

MAKES 1¾ CUPS

---

4 onions, very thinly sliced vertically

¼ cup olive oil

¼ teaspoon kosher salt

⅛ teaspoon freshly ground black pepper

"Sweat" the onions: In a large skillet with a lid, add onions, cover, and cook over medium-low heat for about 20 minutes, stirring every 5 minutes or so to prevent sticking to the pan.

Remove cover and add oil. Continue to cook onions for another 20 minutes or more, stirring about every 5 minutes until onions are browning but not burning. Season with salt and pepper.

USE IN THESE RECIPES

Portabella Mushroom Burgers (p. 127)
Sprouted Wheat Crust Pizza (p. 143)

Frizzled Leeks

A dish with a fun name that's even more fun to eat. You know those crunchy fried onions on green bean casserole? Yup. This recipe is intended to top dishes such as our Roasted Butternut Squash Soup (p. III), but these little leeks are so delicious that you are bound to nibble.

YIELD VARIES

---

1 or more large leeks

1 cup canola or other neutral oil with a high smoke point

⅛ teaspoon kosher salt per leek

USE IN THIS RECIPE

Roasted Butternut Squash Soup (p. 111)

Trim leek, as this recipe uses only the white and very pale green parts. Compost the top. Cut the leek in half lengthwise. Lay halves on your cutting board cut side down and proceed to julienne the leek, also called a "matchstick" cut. You can cut each of the halved leeks into 2-inch sections. Then slice each section into very thin strips. Dry with a clean kitchen towel.

Heat oil in a medium pan over medium heat until very hot. Fry leeks in batches, one handful at a time, separating the thin strips of leek so they cook evenly. Watch closely and remove leeks with a slotted spoon or skimmer when the thin strips are golden brown. This will only take 1–2 minutes at most. Each batch will likely cook more quickly than the last, as the oil will get hotter. Leeks can go from brown to burnt quickly, so watch them carefully.

Once leeks are starting to brown, remove from oil and place on a baking sheet lined with a paper towel to absorb extra oil. Sprinkle with salt while still warm. Spread leeks out in a single layer to cool and crisp.

You can save the oil to use in other recipes, such as frying falafels (p. 146). Our Sautéed Mushrooms Marinated in Garlic (p. 204) or Caramelized Onions (p. 202) call for olive oil, but this extra oil would substitute in well. To save, allow the oil to cool, then transfer to a glass or ceramic container and store in the refrigerator.

Sautéed Mushrooms Marinated in Garlic

These meaty marinated mushrooms are wonderful on pizza, in sandwiches, added to lasagna, and mixed into marinara sauce—that is, if there are enough left over after sampling! If time allows, make these ahead to allow them time to marinate.

MAKES 2 CUPS

1 pound mushrooms, cleaned, trimmed, and sliced

¼ cup olive oil

¼ teaspoon kosher salt

⅛ teaspoon freshly ground black pepper

¼ cup dry white wine (or vermouth) or vegetable broth

2 tablespoons chopped fresh parsley; or 2 teaspoons dried

2 teaspoons minced garlic

In a large nonstick skillet, combine mushrooms, oil, salt, and pepper. Cook over medium heat for about 10 minutes, or until tender. Stir occasionally.

Add cooking wine or broth. Turn up heat to high and cook for 1 minute. Add parsley and garlic. Cook 1 minute more, stirring constantly. Remove from heat. If time allows, let mushrooms marinate at least 1 hour before serving for best flavor.

MAKE IT YOURSELF

Vegetable Broth (p. 293)

USE IN THESE RECIPES

Sprouted Wheat Crust Pizza (p. 143)
Crispy Tofu Parmesan (p. 132)
Foraged Fiddleheads (p. 185)

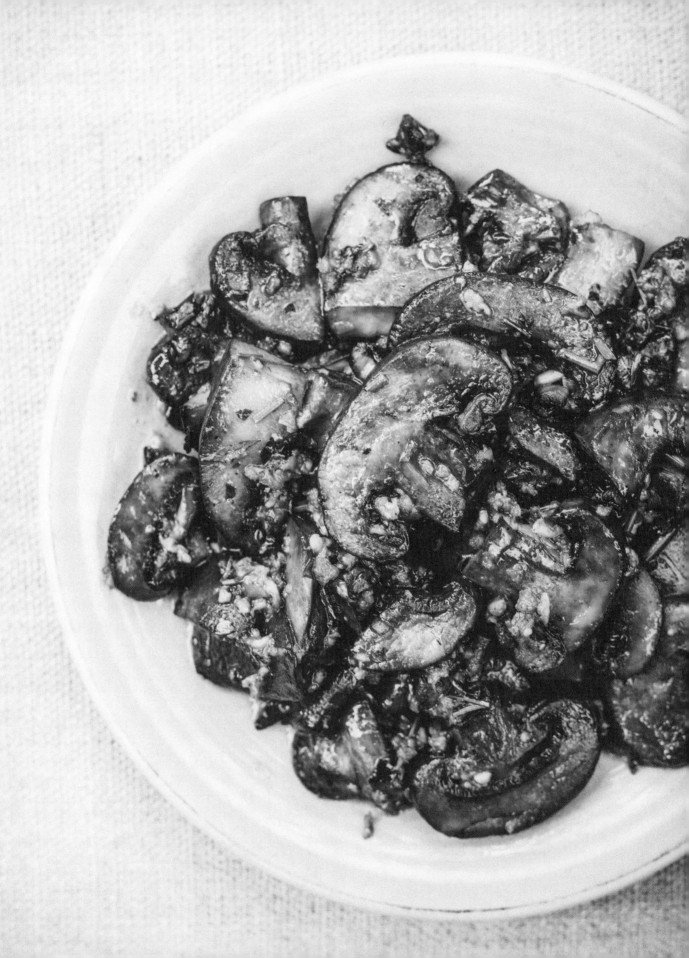

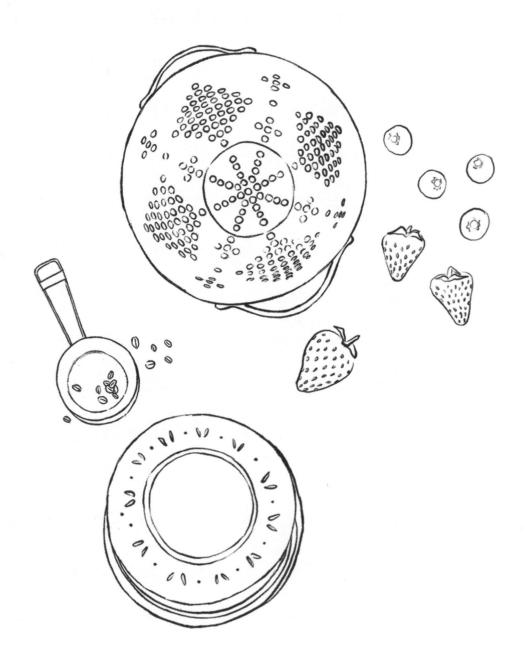

Snacks
and
Sweets

———

Kale Chips

A favorite, especially of kids who may not eat kale in any other form yet will gobble these down. The key to crispy kale is spreading it out in a single layer with no overlapping leaves.

SERVES 4

1 (8-ounce) bunch curly kale

1 tablespoon olive oil

¼ teaspoon salt

Remove and compost kale stems. Tear leaves into chip-sized pieces.

Rinse torn kale leaves and spin in a salad spinner to remove excess water. Use a clean kitchen towel to gently pat dry any remaining moisture from the leaves.

Put kale in a large bowl with the oil. With your hands, gently massage the oil into each leaf until leaves are thoroughly coated.

Spread out kale onto two or three baking sheets in a single layer so leaves are not overlapping. This is the key to crispy kale chips!

Place in a cold oven and turn heat to 300°F. Start timing and bake for about 30 minutes. Stir every 10 minutes. Tongs work well to toss the leaves on their sheets. Each time you stir, rotate the pans in the oven for even cooking—unless you have a convection oven, which automatically circulates the air. Watch closely toward the end of cooking so they don't overcook.

Once crispy, remove from oven. Move all kale chips onto one sheet, sprinkle evenly with salt.

Cool completely. Kale chips will keep their crisp best if left unpackaged at room temperature or put into a paper bag, which allows air to circulate. Re-crisp if needed by placing back in a 300°F oven for 5–10 minutes.

Crispy Roasted Chickpeas

Excellent as a stand-alone snack or as a crunchy topping for salads or soups. These are a healthy alternative to croutons or crackers.

MAKES ¾ CUP

_____

1½ cups cooked chickpeas

1 tablespoon olive oil

1 teaspoon ground cumin

⅛ teaspoon cayenne

¼ teaspoon salt (optional)

Use a clean kitchen towel to pat chickpeas dry. You can remove any chickpea skins that are falling off—this will yield a smoother texture after roasting.

Add chickpeas to a small bowl and toss with oil, cumin, cayenne, and optional salt. Transfer to a baking sheet in a single layer. Place in cold oven and turn heat to 350°F. Start timing and cook for 50 minutes.

To keep crispy, store unpackaged at room temperature if your environment is dry (not humid) for up to several days, or put into a paper bag, which still allows air to circulate. Best enjoyed fresh, so serve soon after roasting.

USE IN THIS RECIPE

Comforting Cauliflower and Potato Soup (p. 112)

Roasted Squash Seeds

Pumpkins aren't the only squash variety with good seeds for roasting. If you are cutting up any winter squash, take the time to clean the seeds and roast them. This cuts back on food waste and uses one of the most nutritious parts of the plant. Seeds are full of fiber, protein, and healthy fats: they are nutrition for nurturing new life. An average pie pumpkin may yield about ½ cup of seeds, so we've based our recipe on that. Adjust the recipe amounts according to how many seeds your squash yields.

MAKES ½ CUP

½ cup fresh squash seeds

¼ teaspoon canola oil

dash salt

Remove seeds from squash. Rinse in water and remove any remaining squash bits and strings. Place on a clean kitchen towel and pat seeds dry.

In a small bowl, mix the clean, dry squash seeds with oil and salt. Spread onto a baking sheet in a single layer.

If you are roasting seeds on their own, place in a cold oven and turn to 350°F. Start timing and roast for about 25 minutes until toasted and golden brown. If even browning is desired, stir about halfway through the cooking time.

If you are roasting the seeds alongside the squash, we call for roasting squash at 450°F, so at this hotter temperature the cook time for the seeds will be reduced to 15 minutes. Make sure to watch the seeds closely and take them out on time to prevent burning.

USE IN THESE RECIPES

Roasted Butternut Squash Soup (p. 111)
Winter Wheat Berry Bowl (p. 149)
Delicata Squash Smiles (p. 194)

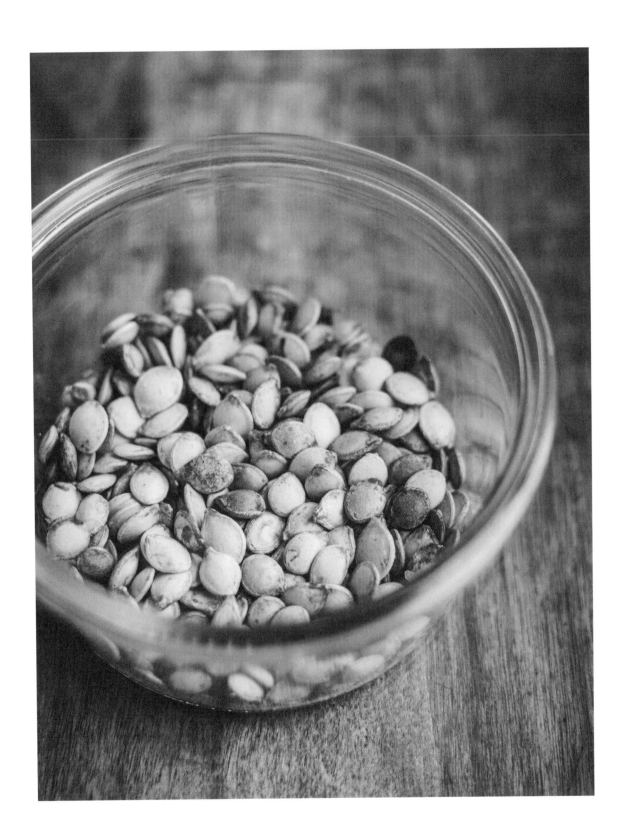

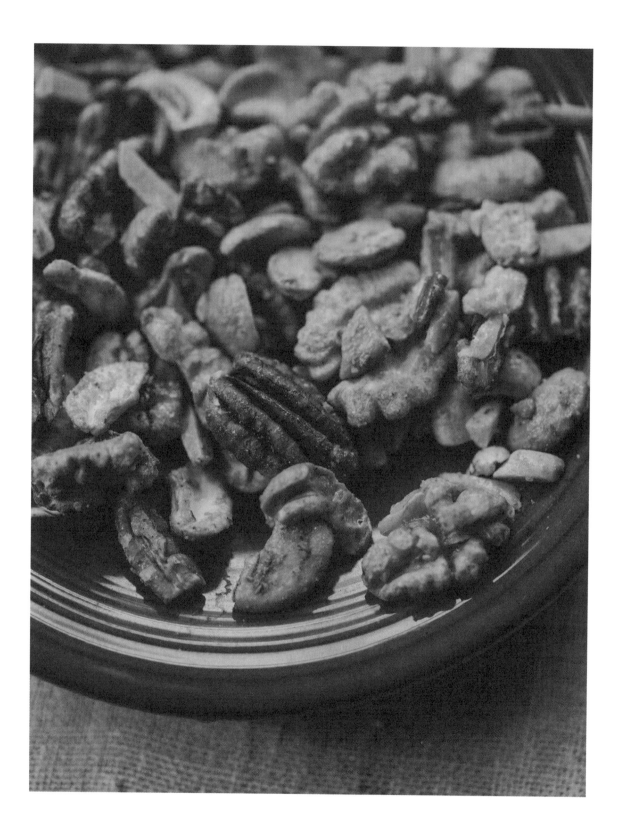

Spiced Nuts

Spice up some nuts with this blend and you'll wow the crowd this holiday or any time of year. Raw nuts are preferable in this recipe, as you are going to be roasting and seasoning them yourself. Walnuts and pecans are typically sold in their raw form. Almonds and cashews can come raw, but are often sold roasted and salted. Use a variety of nuts or pick your favorite. Shelled pistachio nuts add a festive green for the holidays. Brazil nuts, macadamia nuts, and hazelnuts are less common but lovely additions as well.

SERVES 8

2 cups unsalted nuts, any variety or a mix (preferably raw)

1 tablespoon maple syrup

½ teaspoon curry powder

½ teaspoon dried thyme

¼ teaspoon salt

⅛ teaspoon cayenne

Mix all ingredients in a medium bowl until nuts are evenly coated with syrup and spices.

Lightly oil a baking sheet. (Alternatively, for ease of cleanup, line the baking sheet with eco-friendly parchment paper.) Spread nuts out in a single layer.

Place baking sheet in a cold oven and turn to 325°F. Start timing and roast nuts for 20 minutes. Cool completely before serving or storing.

Honey Roasted Peanuts with Popcorn

A sweet and salty snack with satisfying fiber and protein, coming from both the legume (peanuts) and whole grain (popcorn). Double the sauce to turn plain popcorn into caramel corn.

SERVES 8

½ cup popcorn kernels

1 tablespoon butter

2 tablespoons honey

½ teaspoon table salt

½ teaspoon pure vanilla extract (optional)

2 cups shelled unsalted peanuts

⅛ teaspoon kosher salt

MAKE IT YOURSELF

Butter (p. 282)

Pop the popcorn kernels using a method of your choosing: air popper machine, microwave, or stovetop.

To microwave: Place kernels in a brown paper lunch bag, folding top over several times but leaving plenty of space in the bag. Tape flap in place so it stays shut, and microwave on high for 1–2 minutes, until there are several seconds between pops.

To pop on stovetop: Place kernels in a large pot. Add 1 tablespoon canola or other neutral oil. Cover pot and cook over medium heat until most kernels have popped, between 2–4 minutes.

Lightly oil a baking sheet. (Alternatively, line with eco-friendly parchment paper for easy cleanup.)

Melt the butter in a small saucepan. Whisk in the honey, table salt, and optional vanilla, if desired. Add peanuts and stir until evenly coated. Spread nuts out in a single layer on baking sheet.

Place baking sheet in a cold oven and turn to 325°F. Start timing and roast for about 20–25 minutes.

Remove from oven and stir nuts while they are cooling, to break up the clumps and distribute the honey coating. After the nuts have cooled slightly, sprinkle with kosher salt. Cool completely before serving or storing.

Toss popcorn and 1 cup peanuts together. Reserve remaining cup of honey roasted peanuts to combine with another batch of popcorn later, or snack on by themselves. Enjoy fresh. Store any extras in an airtight container.

Caramel corn variation: To transform plain popcorn into caramel corn, make a double batch of the butter and honey sauce. Put popcorn in a big bowl. Pour about half the sauce over the popcorn (the other half goes on the peanuts per the above recipe). Toss the popcorn so it is evenly coated with sauce. Prepare a second baking sheet (oiling it lightly or lining with parchment paper) and spread the popcorn out on the sheet. Bake in the oven along with the peanuts, same temperature and time as above.

Maple Candied Walnuts

These tasty treats celebrate the early spring season in New England. Sap flows from maple trees, providing wild-harvested, organic sweetness for our pleasure. It takes forty gallons of sap to make one gallon of syrup. Thinking about where our food comes from brings joy and appreciation to the eating experience!

SERVES 8

2 cups chopped walnuts halves or pieces

⅓ cup maple syrup

⅛ teaspoon salt

OPTIONAL SEASONING

1 teaspoon ground cinnamon, pure vanilla extract, or cayenne (choose one)

Preheat a nonstick skillet over medium heat.

Add walnuts, syrup, and salt to the skillet. If you are using one of the optional seasonings, add it now.

Cook, stirring constantly, until nuts are toasted and syrup has caramelized, about 3 minutes.

Lightly oil a work surface such as baking sheet, cutting board, or heatproof countertop. (Alternatively, line your work surface with eco-friendly parchment paper or a silicone baking sheet.) Transfer walnuts from skillet to prepared work surface. Separate walnuts so they don't clump together.

Cool completely. For short-term storage, keep in an airtight container at room temperature. For longer shelf life, keep nuts in the refrigerator or freezer.

Serving suggestions: Sprinkle candied walnuts on top of salads, oatmeal, yogurt, muffins, whipped squash, or sweet potatoes. Enjoy a handful for a sweet snack.

USE IN THESE RECIPES

Pear Walnut Salad (p. 69)
Summer Berry and Spinach Salad (p. 71)

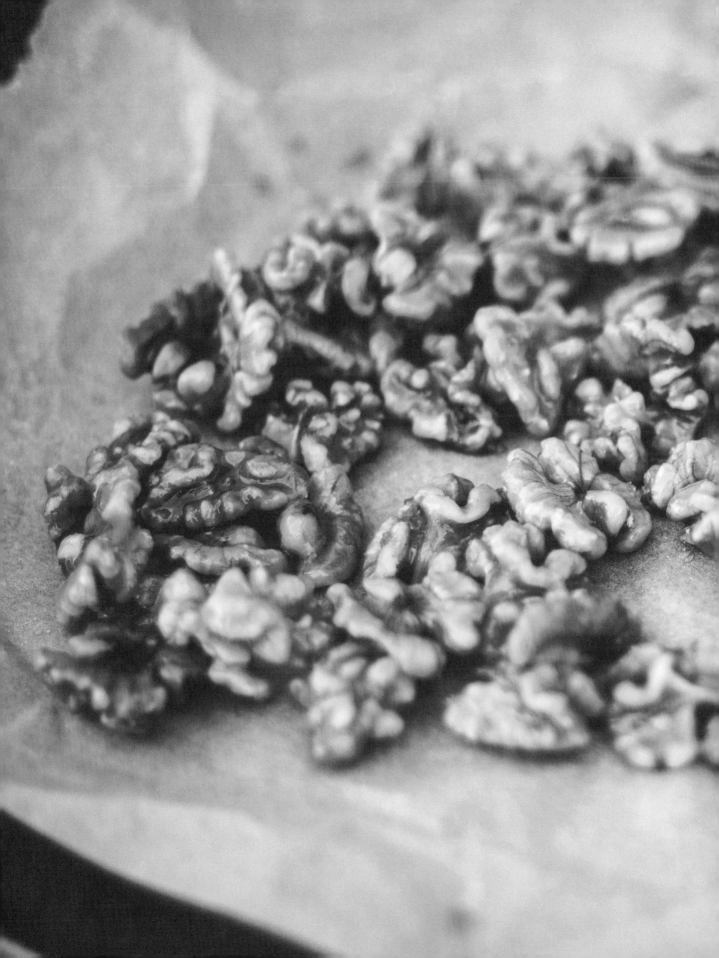

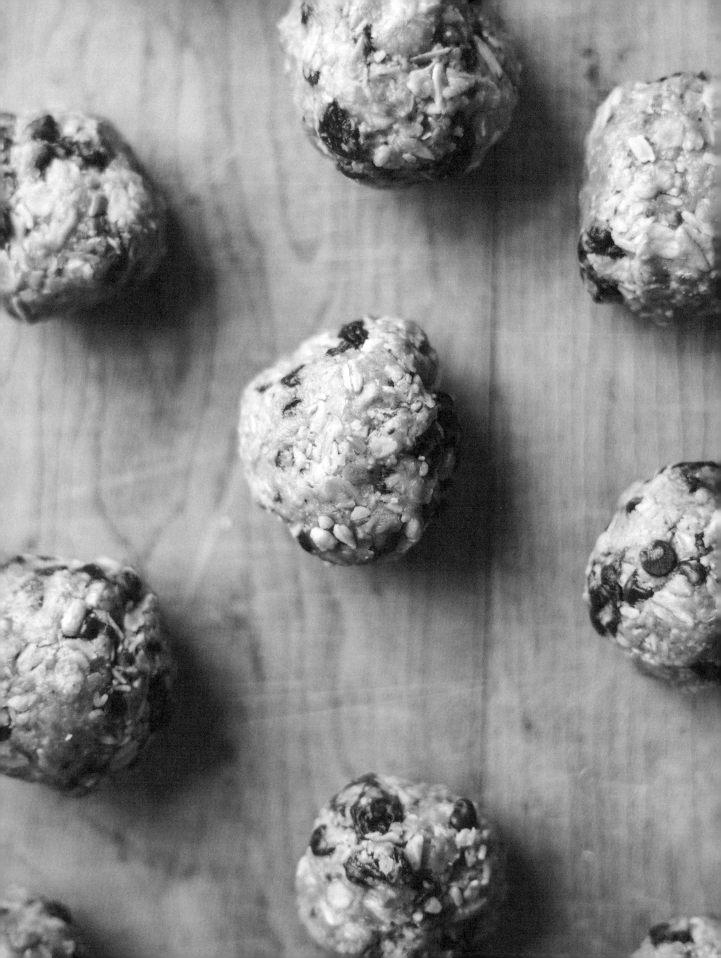

Energy Balls

There is great ease and satisfaction in making these snack-sized bites, especially if that means less consumption of commercial bars, which generate packaging waste. Most of the ingredients have a long shelf life, so consider buying in bulk to further reduce what enters the landfill.

MAKES 24 BALLS

1½ cups rolled oats

1 cup natural nut butter

½ cup shelled sunflower seeds

½ cup unsweetened shredded coconut

½ cup dried cranberries or raisins

⅓–½ cup honey or maple syrup

⅓–½ cup mini chocolate chips

¼ cup freshly ground flaxseed

1 teaspoon pure vanilla extract

Place all ingredients into a food processor. Process until everything starts to come together. Stop to scrape down the insides of the food processor as needed so all ingredients are evenly processed.

Scoop out approximately 2 tablespoons at a time and form into balls. (Alternatively, press into an 8 x 8-inch pan to make bars.)

Refrigerate for at least 30 minutes to firm up before serving. Store in an airtight container in the refrigerator for up to 2 weeks or in the freezer for up to 3 months. We guarantee they will be eaten up before then!

MAKE IT YOURSELF

Natural Nut or Seed Butters (p. 270)

One-of-a-Kind Bars

Customize these bars by using your favorite nuts, seeds, and dried fruits—whatever you happen to have on hand. Seeds may be small, but they are packed with nutrients.

MAKES 16 BARS

1 cup unsweetened shredded coconut

1 cup chopped unsalted nuts (such as almonds, cashews, pistachios, or pecans)

1 cup raw seeds (such as pumpkin, sesame, sunflower, chia, hemp, or poppy seed)

½ cup dried fruit (such as cranberries, cherries, or raisins)

2 tablespoons freshly ground flaxseed

⅛ teaspoon salt

½ cup maple syrup or honey (warmed for easier mixing)

2 tablespoons natural nut or seed butter

1 teaspoon pure vanilla extract (optional)

Mix together all ingredients in a medium bowl until combined.

Oil an 8 x 8-inch baking pan. (Alternatively, place a piece of eco-friendly parchment in the pan, leaving extra paper on all sides for easy removal.)

Pour mixture into pan and, using wet hands or the back of a spoon, spread it out until flat and packed in firmly.

Place in a cold oven and turn to 325°F. Start timing and bake for 20 minutes.

Remove from oven and let cool at room temperature for about 1 hour. Refrigerate for another 30 minutes, as this will help the bars retain their shape when cut.

MAKE IT YOURSELF

Natural Nut or Seed Butters (p. 270)

Berry Sauce or Sorbet

This simple sauce can be served warm with pancakes, waffles, or French toast. Refrigerate to serve with yogurt or if you plan to proceed with making sorbet. A medley of berries (sliced strawberries, raspberries, blueberries, and blackberries) is nice; however, you can also use a single berry.

MAKES 2 CUPS

1 pound fresh or frozen berries, thawed

2 tablespoons maple syrup

1 tablespoon freshly squeezed lemon juice

In a medium saucepan over medium heat, bring berries, syrup, and lemon juice to a boil. Boil for about 5 minutes. Remove from heat and let cool slightly. Serve warm over pancakes, waffles, or French toast. Refrigerate at least several hours before serving over yogurt.

Sorbet variation: This version makes 3 cups and requires using an electric ice cream maker. Make the sauce as above but add 1 cup water and increase maple syrup to ¼ cup and lemon juice to 2 tablespoons. To remove seeds, pass the sauce through a food mill. Once sauce has chilled, prepare sorbet according to your ice cream maker directions. It will take about 25 minutes of churning to go from chilled sauce to sorbet.

Applesauce or Apple Butter

Make this sauce in your style, whether that is basic unsweetened, unspiced, or with all the optional ingredients. Choose varieties of apples that are good for saucing, such as Cortland, McIntosh, or heirloom Yellow Transparent. If you wish, adding a bit of raw beet is a trick that imparts pretty pink color. Continuing to cook the applesauce will concentrate it into apple butter.

MAKES ABOUT 6 CUPS SAUCE OR 3 CUPS APPLE BUTTER

---

5 pounds (½ peck) apples

¾ cup water

3 tablespoons freshly squeezed lemon juice

Optional add-ins

¼ cup shredded beet for pink coloring

¼–½ cup maple syrup

2 teaspoons ground cinnamon

½ teaspoon ground nutmeg

Prepare apples: If you do not have a food mill, core and peel apples. Otherwise, just remove apple stems and slice up, since the food mill will separate out the skins and seeds.

In a Dutch oven or very large saucepot, combine apples, water, lemon juice, and beets, if desired. Bring to a boil over medium heat, then reduce heat and simmer until apples are tender, 15–20 minutes, stirring occasionally. Use a food mill to remove any skins and seeds, then return the sauce to the pot (if you peeled and cored the apples, skip this step). Stir in any remaining optional ingredients you desire, adding maple syrup to desired sweetness. If you are proceeding to make apple butter, mix in maple syrup, cinnamon, and nutmeg.

Apple butter variation: Return the pot of sweetened, spiced sauce to medium-low heat and simmer for about 45 minutes. Stir often. Start checking and stirring more often after 30 minutes, as you don't want the thickening sauce to burn.

Alternatively, if you don't want to be as attentive to a simmering pot that might burn, bake the apple butter, which cooks the sauce at a lower heat for longer time. Pour applesauce into a 9 x 13-inch baking pan. Bake at 325°F for 2 hours, stirring about every 30 minutes. Apple butter is done when volume has reduced by about half.

Serving suggestions for apple butter: Spread onto pancakes, waffles, peanut butter sandwiches, grilled cheese; dollop onto crackers with cheese; stir into oatmeal or yogurt; or enjoy by the spoonful.

Canning: If you have a lot of apples to process, both the applesauce and apple butter can be canned and preserved for up to 1 year. Use the boiling-water method (technique on p. 305–306), processing the applesauce for 15 minutes if using pint jars or 20 minutes for quarts; process pints of apple butter for 15 minutes.

MEAL PLANNING

Mondays are my meal planning day. My routine starts by looking at our calendar and talking as a family about the week ahead. Fridays are our "family fun night" and the girls like to offer up ideas for our dinner.

If I'm going to be later getting home one afternoon, then I want to plan for a quick evening meal or have leftovers.

Next I scan the fridge, freezer, and pantry shelves to see what I have on hand that could be incorporated into meals along with items that should be used up in order to prevent food waste. On a scrap paper from the recycling bin I jot down inspirations and must-use-up ingredients. At the same time I take inventory of staples that need restocking. On a different corner of my scrap paper, I start sketching a grocery list of needed items.

Now it's time to meal plan. Flipping through cooking magazines is a fun way for me to come up with new things to try, and scanning my recipe box reminds me of old favorites to make again. Sometimes when I get stuck for inspiration, it can help to go with a theme such as Taco Tuesday, Fish Friday, Stir-Fry Saturday. I check each meal against the Choose My Plate icon[4] which prompts me to ask questions like: What is the protein-rich food? Will at least half my grains be whole this day? Is roughly 50 percent of each meal colorful, filled with fruits and/or veggies, or do I need to add a side salad, veggie soup, or roasted veggies?

Breakfast and snacks don't vary much for us, so I generally don't plan these. At any given time you can open the freezer and find it filled with our favorite snacks: Energy Balls (p. 219), Spiced Nuts (p. 213) Baked Blueberry Oatmeal Bites (p. 49), and Morning Glory Muffins (p. 63). I make note of anything that needs replenishing.

Now that I have my list, it's off to shop with my reusable bags and refillable jars!

Heather

Cranberry Sauce

Use this spiced sauce as a seasonal side to roasted vegetables or as a spread on a sandwich. Add a scoop to a fall Pear Walnut Salad (p. 69) or sprinkle with our Simple Granola (p. 50) for dessert. If you have a leftover spice sachet from mulling cider, you can use that in place of the cinnamon, allspice, and cloves.

MAKES 2 CUPS

---

12 ounces fresh or frozen cranberries

½ cup orange juice, apple cider, or Mulled Apple Cider (p. 240)

½ cup maple syrup, honey, or a combination

¼ cup water

1 stick cinnamon; or ½ teaspoon ground

1 whole allspice; or ¼ teaspoon ground

⅛ teaspoon ground cloves

1 small apple, cored and finely chopped (optional)

½ cup golden or regular raisins or chopped dried apricots (optional)

Put all ingredients, including any optional ones, in a saucepan over medium heat. Bring to a boil, then reduce heat and simmer for at least 10 minutes, or until sauce starts to thicken. Stir occasionally. Remove from heat. If you used any whole spices, remove and compost them. Allow to cool completely before serving.

Pumpkin Spice Dip

This delicious dip comes together quickly for a fall appetizer or dessert. If you like a thick consistency, use cream cheese plus the optional peanut butter.

SERVES 6

½ cup (4 ounces) cream cheese or plain Greek yogurt

¼ cup plain pumpkin puree

2 tablespoons maple syrup

½ teaspoon pure vanilla extract

½ teaspoon ground cinnamon

2 tablespoons peanut butter or other nut or seed butter (optional)

Blend all ingredients together until creamy. You can do this by hand; if you prefer a whipped consistency, use a food processor or blender.

Serving suggestions: Serve with apple slices, celery sticks, or graham crackers.

MAKE IT YOURSELF

Yogurt or Greek Yogurt (p. 280–281)
Natural Nut or Seed Butters (p. 270)

Cran-Apple Crisp

This seasonal treat is tart, with just enough maple syrup to sweeten those cranberries. Feel free to increase the amount of maple syrup if your taste preferences are on the sweeter side.

SERVES 8

8-12 ounces fresh cranberries (2-3 cups)

4 apples, unpeeled, cored, and diced (about 4 cups)

½ cup maple syrup, divided

1 cup rolled oats

½ cup flour (any kind)

½ teaspoon ground cinnamon

⅛ teaspoon table salt

4 tablespoons butter or canola oil

¼ cup finely chopped walnuts or pecans

In an 8 x 8-inch baking pan, mix together cranberries, apples, and ¼ cup maple syrup.

In a separate bowl, mix together oats, flour, cinnamon, and salt. Cut in butter until mixture is crumbly. You can use a pastry cutter, two knives, a fork, or your fingers to incorporate the butter. Add walnuts and the remaining ¼ cup maple syrup. Mix until well combined.

Sprinkle the oat topping over the cranberry-apple filling.

Place in a cold oven and turn to 375°F. Start timing and bake for 35 minutes, or until apples have softened and oat topping is just starting to brown. If apples aren't quite done when the timer goes off, turn off the oven and leave the crisp in the oven for a while longer, as it will retain plenty of heat for continued cooking.

Best served at room temperature as it will set up as it cools.

MAKE IT YOURSELF

Butter (p. 282)

Strawberry-Rhubarb Compote

Rhubarb, an early spring perennial vegetable, is tart and pairs well with sweet strawberries for a classic dessert combination. Compote, a thick sauce, can be eaten many ways: on its own with a sprinkle of granola; mixed into yogurt; as a topping on pancakes, waffles, or French toast; or as the base for a crisp. With all the rhubarb that abounds, make extra and freeze individual portions in ice cube trays. Once frozen, pop out and store in freezer bags, where they will remain available so you can enjoy seasonal compote year-round.

MAKES 2 CUPS

2 cups chopped rhubarb

2 cups hulled and chopped strawberries

¼ cup honey or maple syrup

Combine rhubarb, strawberries, and honey in a medium saucepan over low heat. Stir frequently, cooking until the rhubarb begins to fall apart and the strawberries have softened, about 10 minutes. Taste and sweeten more if desired. Keep in mind that the tart taste of rhubarb is part of what makes it a special spring tonic.

Rhubarb-only variation: To make a rhubarb-only compote, use 4 cups chopped rhubarb and omit the strawberries.

Lebanese Labneh

Labneh is a Middle Eastern yogurt cheese with similarities to cream cheese: it is thick, creamy, and spreadable. It is traditionally served with a drizzle of olive oil and sprinkling of za'atar, a Middle Eastern herb-spice blend, along with pita bread.

MAKES 2-3 CUPS

4 cups (1 quart) plain regular or Greek yogurt

¾ teaspoon table salt

juice of ½ lemon (optional)

OPTIONAL GARNISHES

extra-virgin olive oil for drizzling

za'atar for garnish

MAKE IT YOURSELF

Yogurt or Greek Yogurt (p. 280–281)

NOTE: Full-fat and Greek yogurts will yield the thickest labneh. Regular yogurt will drain off more whey than Greek, yielding about 2 cups labneh from regular and 3 cups from Greek.

Mix together yogurt, salt, and lemon juice, if desired. Place a colander or fine-mesh sieve over a bowl large enough that the colander or sieve doesn't touch the bottom of the bowl. Line the colander or sieve with a thin cotton cloth, such as a clean flour sack towel. Carefully spoon or pour the yogurt mixture into the colander or sieve. Use the overhanging edges of the towel or cloth to cover the yogurt, then refrigerate for 12–24 hours. The longer it drains, the thicker it will be.

When yogurt is done draining, unfold the towel or cloth and either dump or spoon the yogurt into a bowl. For a whipped texture, stir vigorously with a fork.

Scoop ½–1 cup labneh into a serving dish and drizzle oil over the top and sprinkle with za'atar.

Use labneh as you would plain cream cheese. Try it on our Loaded Veggie Sandwich (p. 120), in the Lemon Dill Spinach Artichoke Dip (p. 258), or Summer Berry Yogurt Cheese 'Cake' Parfait (p. 229).

Stored in an airtight container, labneh will last for up to 1 week in the refrigerator.

Summer Berry Yogurt Cheese "Cake" Parfait

We've taken the labneh (yogurt cheese) and created a delicious cheesecake-like dessert by pairing it with our berry sauce. Be sure to make the labneh at least a day ahead, as it takes 12–24 hours to drain. A longer draining time will yield less labneh, hence the volume range below.

SERVES 4-6

2-3 cups Lebanese Labneh (p. 228)

2 cups Berry Sauce (p. 221), chilled

zest of 1 lemon for garnish

Layer in order of labneh-berry sauce-labneh to create a parfait, or spoon berry sauce atop labneh. Garnish with lemon zest if desired.

Aquafaba Meringue Cookies

Who knew the liquid you drain off beans (aquafaba) could produce meringue equal in quality and taste to that of egg-white meringue? Aquafaba from canned low sodium white beans yields by far the best results. This is a great treat to whip up after making any of our many recipes that call for chickpeas.

MAKES 40 MERINGUES

⅔–¾ cup canned chickpea or cannelini bean aquafaba, at room temperature

¼ teaspoon cream of tartar

1 teaspoon pure vanilla extract

⅓ cup granulated maple sugar (not syrup)

NOTE: In our recipe testing, aquafaba from canned beans made, by far, the best meringue. Aquafaba from dried, soaked, and cooked beans took longer to create stiff peaks (if at all) and didn't hold form as well during baking. Preferably, aquafaba should come from no added salt or low sodium chickpeas. One (15½-ounce) can provides the amount of aquafaba needed for this recipe.

In a stand mixer with whisk attachment, beat aquafaba and cream of tartar on high speed until stiff peaks form, about 6 minutes.

While still beating, add vanilla and then the sugar, about 1 tablespoon at a time, stopping to scrape down the sides if needed.

Line two baking sheets with eco-friendly parchment paper. Drop 1 heaping tablespoon meringue onto baking sheet in a mound. Repeat.

Place in a cold oven and turn to 200°F. Bake until completely dry to the touch, about 2 hours. Rotate the pans halfway through the cooking time. Turn oven off and let meringues sit in the oven for 1 hour or so; the residual heat will continue drying out the inside center of the meringues.

Cool completely before serving or storing in an airtight container. Will store up to 5 days.

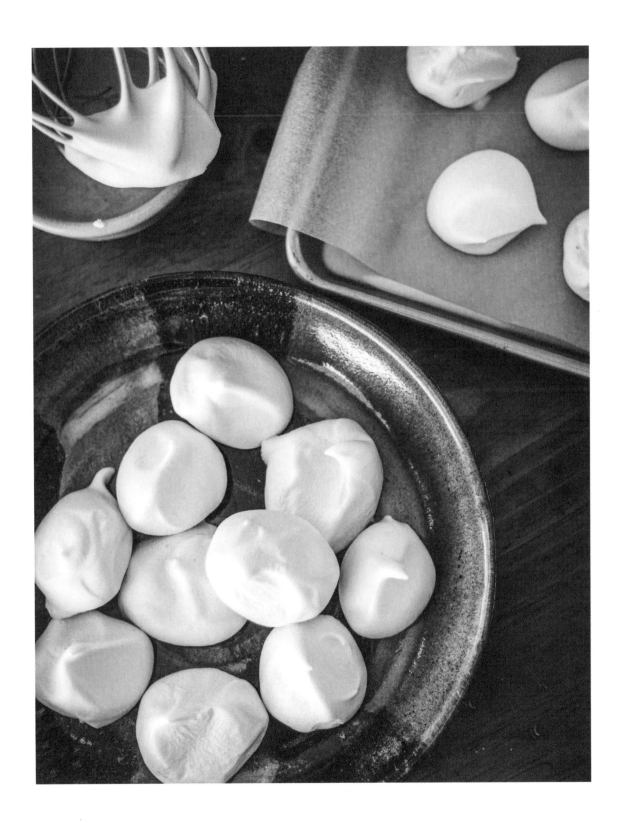

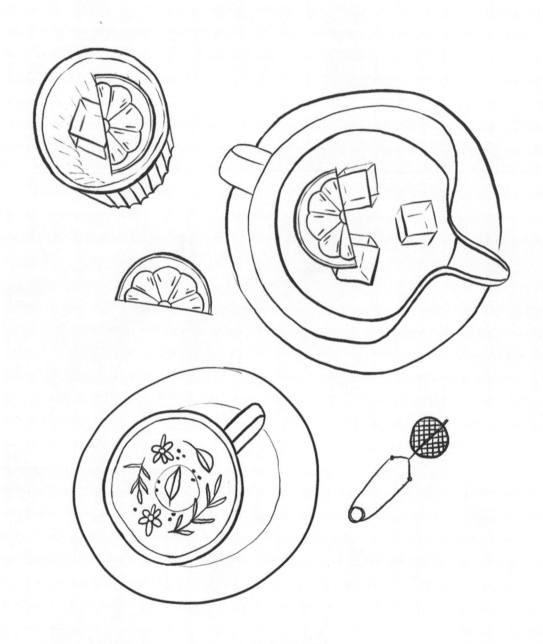

Drinks

———

Herb-Infused Cucumber Lemon Water

There are endless flavor combinations that add interest to water without calories. This refreshing infusion calls for cucumber, citrus, and two herbs: rosemary and mint.

SERVES 8

---

8 cups water

6 (2- to 3-inch) sprigs fresh rosemary

6 (2- to 3-inch) sprigs fresh mint

1 lemon, sliced into thin rounds

1 small cucumber, sliced into thin rounds

Measure water into a pitcher.

Wash herbs. Roll herbs gently between your hands to crush slightly, releasing their fragrance.

Add herbs, lemon, and cucumber to the water. To infuse, refrigerate for at least 1 hour or as long as overnight.

After you've finished this first infusion, you can reuse the herbs, lemon and cucumber for a second infusion if desired.

Watermelon Basil Water

If you find you have more watermelon than you can possible eat by the slice, blend up extra into a basil-infused beverage. Watermelon is more than 90 percent water by weight, so you'll have no trouble staying hydrated with this refreshing summertime drink.

SERVES 8

---

8 cups seedless watermelon chunks

2 cups water

juice of 2 limes

½ cup fresh basil

Add watermelon, water, and lime juice to a blender. Blend until smooth. There will be very little pulp left. If you prefer no pulp, strain through a fine-mesh sieve, pushing the liquid through with the help of a spoon, swirling and pressing the watermelon water into a bowl.

Wash basil. Roll the basil gently between your hands to crush slightly, releasing its fragrance.

Add basil to the watermelon water. To infuse, refrigerate for at least 1 hour or as long as overnight.

Berry Banana Smoothie

This smoothie combines probiotics (good bacteria) from the yogurt with prebiotics (non-digestible soluble fibers that pass through the gastrointestinal tract and act as food for the probiotics). Bananas, berries, ground flaxseed, and oats are all good sources of prebiotic fibers.

SERVES 2

---

1 frozen or fresh banana

1 cup frozen or fresh berries

¾ cup yogurt

¼ cup milk

¼ cup rolled oats

2 tablespoons freshly ground flaxseed

1 tablespoon honey or maple syrup (optional)

MAKE IT YOURSELF

Yogurt or Greek Yogurt (p. 280–281)

Place all ingredients in blender. Blend until well combined. Add more milk if you want a thinner smoothie.

NOTE: Berry seeds, ground flaxseed, and oats will maintain some texture even after blending, so this smoothie will not have a completely smooth mouthfeel. If leftover smoothie sits, it will thicken as the soluble oats soak up liquid. It may be necessary to thin any leftover mixture with a splash of milk.

NOTE: If you want to try kefir (a fermented milk drink similar to drinkable yogurt), substitute 1 cup kefir in place of the yogurt and milk.

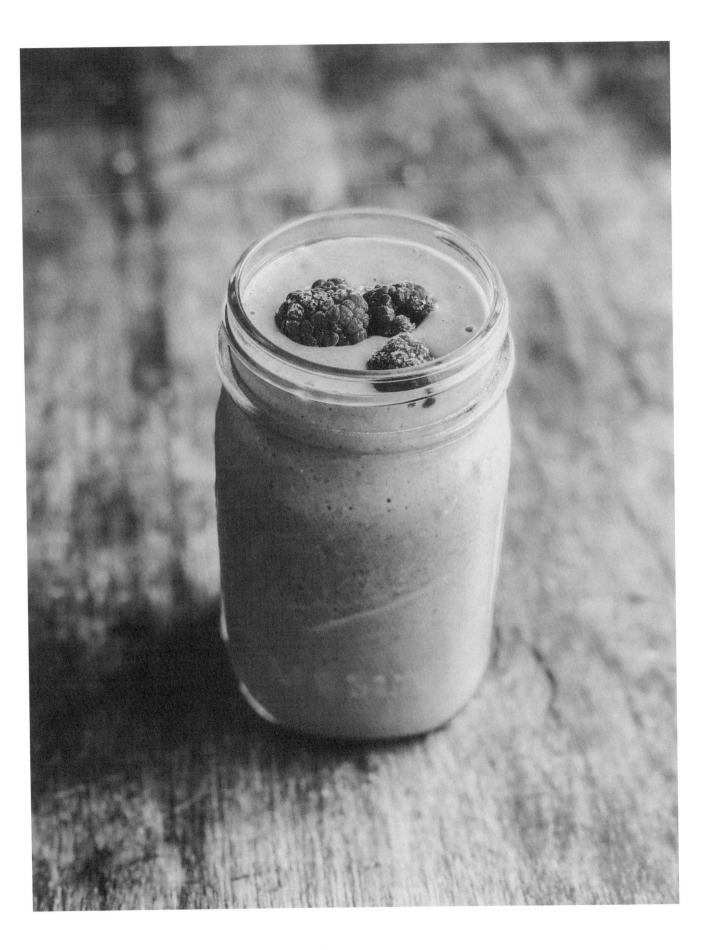

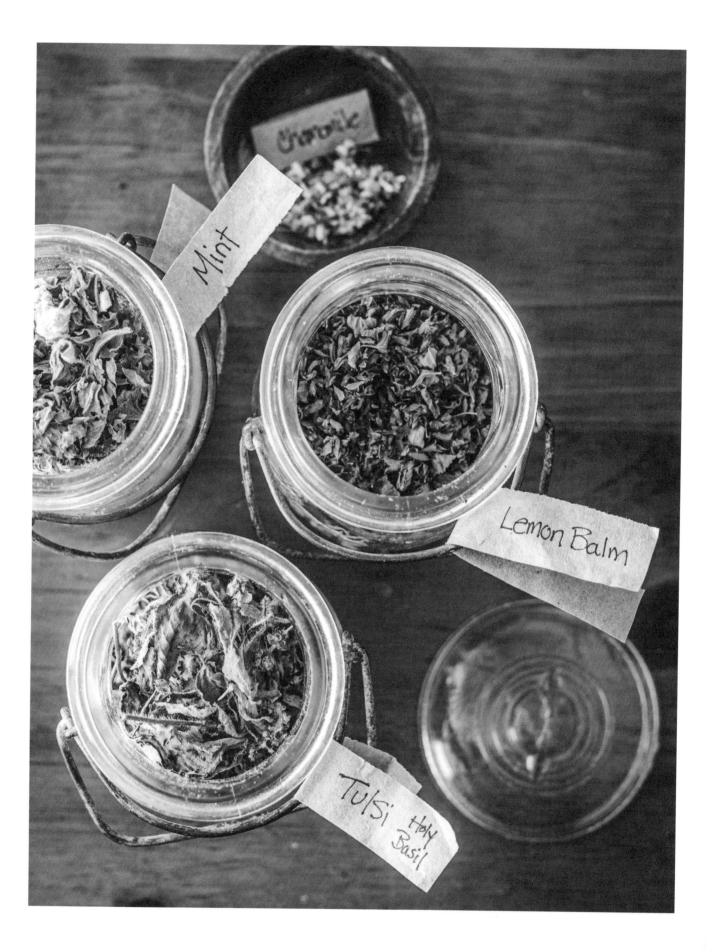

Restorative Herbal Tea

Drinking tea is restorative to body and soul. Herbs have been used as a healing remedy since ancient times. This is an herbal blend of medicinal nervines (calming) and adaptogens (balancing). Get an added therapeutic benefit when you grow your own herbs. Tulsi, or holy basil, is a favorite adaptogen that makes delicious tea. It is a warm weather annual that must be started indoors and then transplanted into the garden. You can also substitute culinary sweet basil.

MAKES 4 CUPS

---

2 tablespoons dried mint leaves; or ¼ cup fresh

2 tablespoons dried holy basil (tulsi) leaves; or ¼ cup fresh

2 tablespoons dried lemon balm leaves; or ¼ cup fresh

½ teaspoon dried chamomile flowers; or 1 teaspoon fresh (optional)

4 cups boiling water

Place herbs in a clean, empty glass quart jar. Fill the jar with boiling water, covering the herbs. Steep the tea for about 30 minutes. Use a fine-mesh sieve to strain. You can refill the jar for a second infusion reusing the same herbs. It will yield a slightly weaker but worthwhile brew.

You can enjoy this tea hot, at room temperature, or chilled. Reheat as needed. Store extra at room temperature for up to 1 day or refrigerate up to 1 week.

Iced tea variation: Make a double strong infusion by using the recipe above, but decreasing water to 2 cups. After the concentrated tea has finished steeping and been strained, add enough ice cubes to double the volume of liquid, bringing the total volume up to 4 cups. Stir in ice to chill. Refrigerate if serving later. Garnish with fresh mint and lemon slices if desired.

Mulled Apple Cider

Serving a comforting cup of warm apple cider that has been mulled with spices is just the ticket for an autumnal gathering. You can easily scale down the portions to make less.

SERVES 16

---

6 sticks cinnamon

1 tablespoon whole allspice

1 tablespoon whole cloves plus 1 teaspoon for garnish

1 gallon apple cider

1 large orange, cut into 16 half slices, for garnish

Make a sachet of the spices using cheesecloth and kitchen string: put cinnamon sticks, allspice, and 1 tablespoon cloves in the center of a cheesecloth square, pull up the four corners, and tie with kitchen string. Alternatively, add the spices loose and strain them out later, or the allspice and cloves could go into a tea ball infuser.

Pour cider into a large saucepan or soup pot. Add the spices, either packaged or loose. Bring to a boil. Cover, reduce heat, and simmer for 20 minutes.

Strain the cider to remove any loose spices.

Optional garnish: Stick 1 teaspoon whole cloves into the rind of the orange slices. Serve cider with clove-studded orange slices. These can be floated in the large saucepan or placed individually in each cup.

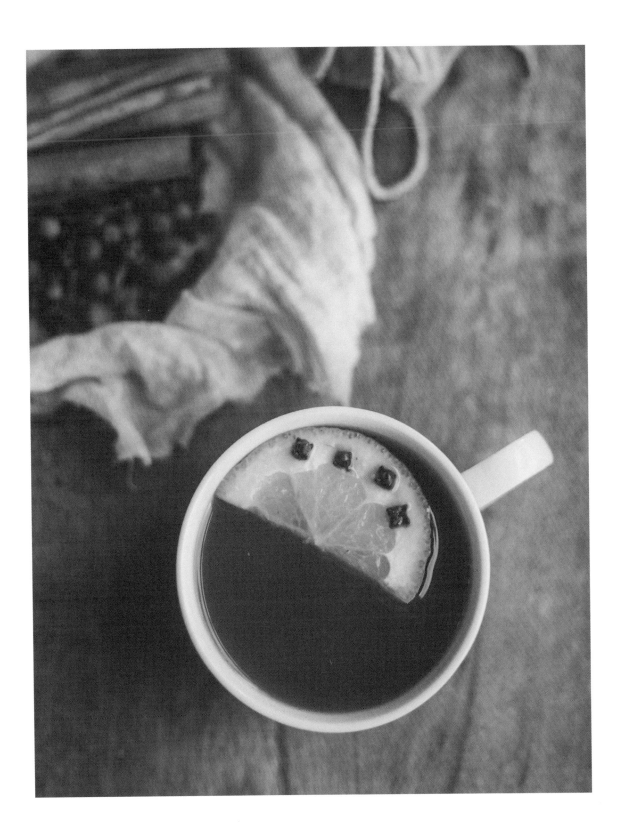

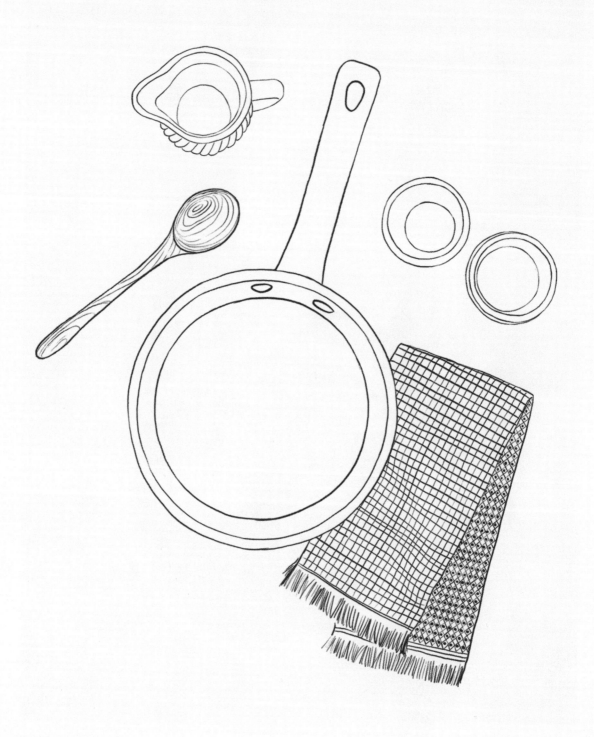

Sauces, Dips, and Dressings

Marinara Sauce

A simple, homemade tomato sauce that has no added sugars, is low in sodium, and is full of flavor. Use fresh tomatoes in season and canned tomatoes other times of year (be sure to recycle the can).

MAKES 3 CUPS

---

1 tablespoon olive oil

½ cup finely chopped onion

3 cloves garlic, minced

2 pounds fresh tomatoes, cored and diced (about 4 cups); or 1 (28-ounce) can diced, crushed, or pureed

½ teaspoon kosher salt

1 tablespoon minced fresh oregano; or 1 teaspoon dried

1 tablespoon minced fresh basil; or 1 teaspoon dried

1 tablespoon minced fresh parsley; or 1 teaspoon dried

Add oil to a saucepan and sauté onions over medium-high heat until softened, about 5 minutes. Add garlic and cook another minute. Add tomatoes and salt. Season with oregano, basil, and parsley.

Simmer 30 minutes over low heat. Enjoy chunky, or if you prefer a smooth sauce, blend or puree (technique on p. 307). The sauce can also be put through a food mill to remove skins and seeds if desired; however, these are edible and nutritious components to include if you don't mind them.

USE IN THESE RECIPES

Crispy Tofu Parmesan with Sautéed Mushrooms (p. 132)
Sprouted Wheat Crust Pizza (p. 143)

MAKE IT YOURSELF

Canned Diced Tomatoes (p. 274)

Enchilada Sauce

The same basic sauce as our marinara, except spiced differently.

MAKES 3 CUPS

1 tablespoon olive oil

½ cup finely chopped onion

3 cloves garlic, minced

1 tablespoon chili powder

1 teaspoon ground cumin

2 pounds fresh tomatoes, cored and diced (about 4 cups); or 1 (28-ounce) can diced, crushed, or pureed

½ teaspoon kosher salt

2 teaspoons honey (optional)

Add oil to a saucepan and sauté onions over medium-high heat until softened, about 5 minutes. Add garlic, chili powder, and cumin and cook another minute. Add tomatoes, salt, and optional honey.

Simmer 30 minutes over low heat. Enjoy chunky, or if you prefer a smooth sauce, blend or puree (technique on p. 307). The sauce can also be put through a food mill to remove skins and seeds if desired; however, these are edible and nutritious components.

USE IN THESE RECIPES

Three Sisters Succotash Enchiladas (p. 178)
Sweet Potato and Black Bean Enchiladas (p. 177)
Quinoa Enchilada Skillet (p. 169)

MAKE IT YOURSELF

Canned Diced Tomatoes (p. 274)

LEARNING TO EAT AT HOME

Moves are never easy. When we transitioned to life in Vermont, it meant going from city life to rural life, from renting to owning a home, and from flat land to mountains. Very early on, when all our kitchen items were in boxes and our refrigerator and pantry were not yet stocked, we quickly learned that eating dinner out was pretty much impossible unless we were willing to drive thirty minutes one way. All the restaurants near us closed by late afternoon or were closed for the entire winter season. We realized that everyone in the area eats dinner at home most of the time, so restaurants can't afford to be open for dinner. This truth, which annoyed me at the time, became something I am now grateful for. It has pushed our family to have dinners planned and our kitchen stocked. We still sometimes grab takeout from our favorite Indian or Chinese restaurant, but we have learned to lean less on restaurants to fill the gaps.

Classic Basil Pesto

Basil pesto can be used for many things. A spoonful or two can flavor cooked whole grains or roasted veggies, serve as the sauce on a white pizza or a sandwich spread, be stirred into a white bean veggie soup or ratatouille, or serve as a topping for crackers or a dip for crudité.

MAKES 1 CUP

¼ cup pine nuts or chopped walnuts

2 packed cups fresh basil

¼ cup freshly grated Parmesan cheese

1 large clove garlic, minced

3 tablespoons extra-virgin olive oil

2 tablespoons water

¼ teaspoon kosher salt

⅛ teaspoon freshly ground black pepper

Toast the nuts (technique on p. 312). Toasting nuts improves flavor and texture and only takes a few minutes.

Add all the ingredients into a food processor and process until desired consistency is achieved. Pause to scrape down sides of bowl as needed. You can use a small amount of additional water to make the consistency thinner.

If you're not going to use up pesto within the week, you can freeze it to use later. Use ice cube trays to freeze single servings. Once frozen, pop the cubes out and store in labeled and dated freezer bags.

USE IN THESE RECIPES

Edamame Caprese Salad (p. 84)

Caprese Grilled Cheese (p. 118)

Spring Veggie and Pesto Pasta (p. 137)

Sprouted Wheat Crust Pizza (p. 143)

Roasted Veggies for All Seasons, spring variation (p. 192)

Carrot Top Pesto

Carrot tops shall never again be discarded as food waste once you've tried this recipe. Freeze any extra pesto in ice cube trays and store in freezer bags for use anytime. Try using other greens, such as arugula, beet greens, chard, or kale, in place of carrot tops.

MAKES 1 CUP

¼ cup walnuts, pecans, or pine nuts

2 cups carrot tops, chopped (tops from 4-5 large carrots)

2 cloves garlic, minced

½ cup fresh basil (optional)

⅓ cup extra-virgin olive oil

¼ cup freshly grated Parmesan cheese

¼ teaspoon kosher salt

⅛ teaspoon freshly ground black pepper

water to thin, as desired

Toast the nuts (technique on p. 312). Toasting nuts improves flavor and texture, and only takes a few minutes.

In the bowl of a food processor, add nuts, carrot tops, garlic, optional basil, oil, Parmesan cheese, salt, and pepper. Process until ingredients are well combined. Stop to scrape down sides as needed. Add water, 1 tablespoon at a time, until desired consistency is achieved.

Serve as you would any pesto.

USE IN THESE RECIPES

Spice-Rubbed Roasted Carrots (p. 191)
Any recipe that calls for Classic Basil Pesto (p. 247)

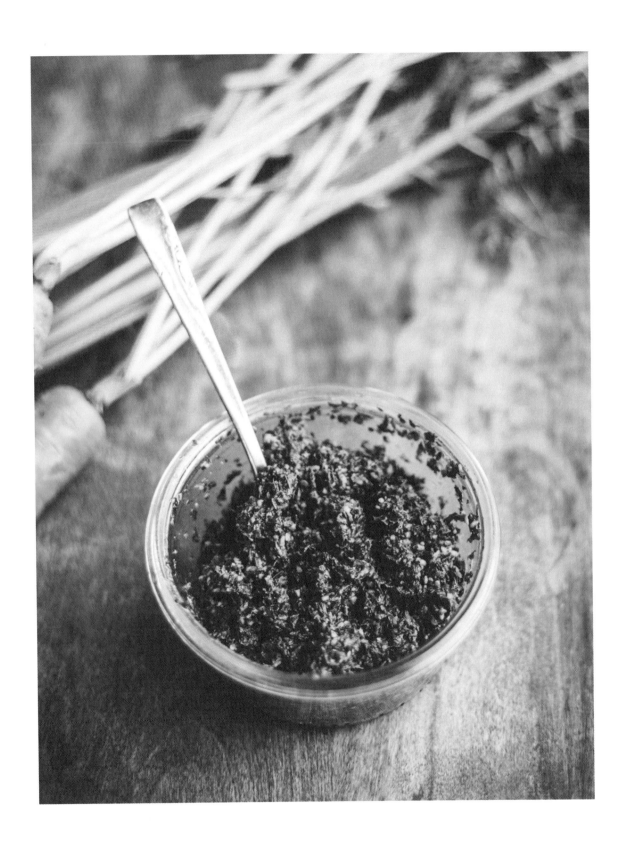

Classic Tzatziki

Tzatziki is a yogurt-cucumber-garlic sauce of Greek origin. Ideally, mix this recipe at least an hour before you plan to serve it, which will allow time for the flavors to meld in the refrigerator.

MAKES 1½ CUPS

1 cup grated cucumber (see recipe instructions)

1 cup plain Greek yogurt

1-2 cloves garlic, minced

1 tablespoon chopped fresh dill weed; or 1 teaspoon dried

1 tablespoon freshly squeezed lemon juice

1 tablespoon extra-virgin olive oil

¼ teaspoon kosher salt

Prepare cucumber: Seeding and peeling is recommended if using bigger, older cucumbers but unnecessary if cucumbers are small, young, or seedless. Grate cucumber. As an optional step, remove excess water by either squeezing the grated cucumber in your hands over the sink, pressing it in a clean kitchen towel, or lightly salting and letting it sit in a colander in the sink for about 30 minutes.

Combine cucumber with remaining ingredients, stirring until well mixed.

Refrigerate until ready to serve. For best flavor, refrigerate at least 1 hour before serving.

USE IN THESE RECIPES

Falafel (p. 146)

MAKE IT YOURSELF

Greek Yogurt (p. 280–281)

Classic Hummus

This classic chickpea-tahini hummus contains fiber and protein that will satisfy as a snack on whole grain crackers, as a dip for veggies, as a scoop added to a salad, or as a spread on sandwiches. Add interest to classic hummus by adding ingredients such as this nicely spiced roasted red pepper version.

MAKES 2 CUPS

¼ cup tahini

juice of 1 lemon

2 tablespoons extra-virgin olive oil

1-2 cloves garlic, minced

½ teaspoon kosher salt

1½ cups cooked chickpeas

water or aquafaba, to thin

ADDITIONAL INGREDIENTS FOR ROASTED RED PEPPER HUMMUS

½ teaspoon ground cumin

¼ teaspoon cayenne

¾ cup (7 ounces) chopped roasted red peppers

Combine tahini and lemon juice in a food processor or blender. Process for approximately 1 minute.

Add oil, garlic, and salt. Process for another minute.

Add chickpeas and continue to process until smooth, adding water 1 tablespoon at a time until the hummus is your desired consistency.

Store homemade hummus in an airtight container and refrigerate up to 1 week.

Roasted red pepper variation: Prepare hummus as above, but add cumin and cayenne when adding oil, garlic, and salt. Add roasted red peppers when adding chickpeas.

MAKE IT YOURSELF

Tahini (p. 273)

Roasted Red Peppers (p. 275)

USE IN THESE RECIPES

Roasted Beet and Goat Cheese Sandwich (p. 70)

Greek Cucumber Chopped Salad (p. 80)

Crunchy Hummus Veggie Wrap (p. 123)

Antipasto Platter or Sandwich (p. 119)

Falafel (p. 146)

Roasted Veggie and Chickpea Bowl (p. 150)

Peanut Sauce

Peanuts are an atypical legume crop in that the pod actually develops underground. The oily, edible seeds we enjoy eating are harvested from these pods. This versatile peanut sauce is used to add Asian fusion flavors to several of our recipes. It can be served thicker or thinner, depending on how much water you add. If you love peanut sauce, we recommend doubling the recipe!

MAKES ½ CUP

¼ cup natural peanut butter

juice of ½ lime

2 tablespoons reduced sodium tamari or soy sauce

1 tablespoon water plus additional to thin

2 teaspoons honey

1 teaspoon minced or grated fresh ginger; or ⅓ teaspoon ground

½ teaspoon minced garlic

¼ teaspoon sriracha hot chili sauce or hot red pepper flakes

Whisk all ingredients in a small bowl or shake them together in a jar with a tight-fitting lid.

If a thinner sauce is desired, add more water, 1 tablespoon at a time, until desired consistency is achieved.

USE IN THESE RECIPES

Bow "Thai" Salad (p. 93)
Thai Veggie Tofu Wrap (p. 117)
Thai Veggie Brown Rice Bowl (p. 165)

MAKE IT YOURSELF

Natural Nut Butter (p. 270)

Raita

Raita, an Indian yogurt-cucumber sauce, is served to counter the heat of spicy dishes. Pair this with one of the recipes suggested below or with your favorite curry dish.

MAKES 1½ CUPS

½ cup grated cucumber (see recipe instructions)

1 cup plain Greek yogurt

¼ teaspoon ground cumin

¼ teaspoon kosher salt

OPTIONAL ADD-INS

2 tablespoons chopped fresh cilantro or mint

2 tablespoons chopped red onion or green onions

1 tablespoon freshly squeezed lemon or lime juice

Prepare cucumber: Seeding and peeling is recommended if using bigger, older cucumbers but unnecessary if cucumbers are small, young, or seedless. Grate cucumber. As an optional step, remove excess water by either squeezing the grated cucumber in your hands over the sink, pressing it in a clean kitchen towel, or lightly salting and letting it sit in a colander in the sink for about 30 minutes.

Combine all main ingredients and any desired optional add-ins in a medium bowl.

Refrigerate until ready to serve. For best flavor, refrigerate at least 1 hour before serving.

USE IN THESE RECIPES

Red Lentil Dhal (p. 159)
Gobi Masala (p. 156)

MAKE IT YOURSELF

Greek Yogurt (p. 280–281)

Fresh Salsa

When tomatoes are ripe, make salsa! Quick, easy, and so fresh. There is no substitute for fresh salsa, and it's worth the extra five minutes to combine these fresh ingredients to take your meals to the next level. Because the ingredients are fresh, this salsa can be kept in an airtight container in the refrigerator for no longer than five days. Roma tomatoes are recommended; leave jalapeño seeds in for a hotter spice level.

MAKES 3 CUPS

3 tomatoes, quartered

½ jalapeño pepper, seeded and roughly chopped

½ small onion (not sweet), quartered

2 cloves garlic, chopped or minced

½ loosely packed cup fresh cilantro

juice of ½ lime

¼ teaspoon kosher salt

dash ground cumin

Place all ingredients in a blender or food processor and pulse, making sure the mixture is still chunky and not pureed. Taste and adjust seasonings if desired. Refrigerate at least 1 hour. The salsa may be lighter red than store-bought salsa, although it may darken with time.

USE IN THESE RECIPES

Breakfast Tacos (p. 46)

Tomato Gazpacho (p. 113)

Seven-Layer Burrito Pan (p. 173)

Chorizo Quesadillas (p. 174)

Guacamole (p. 257)

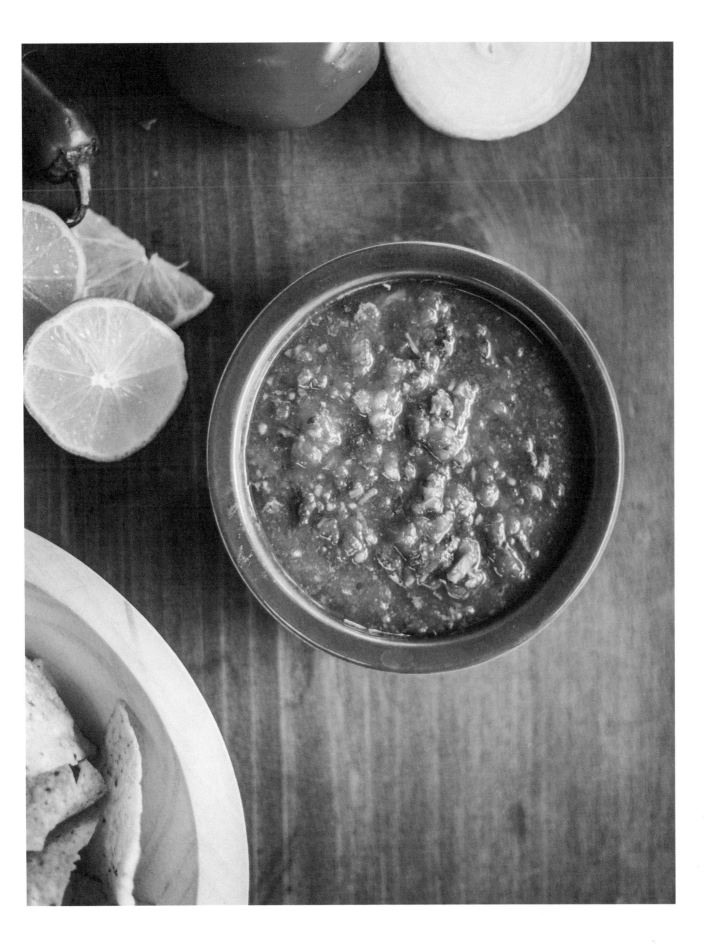

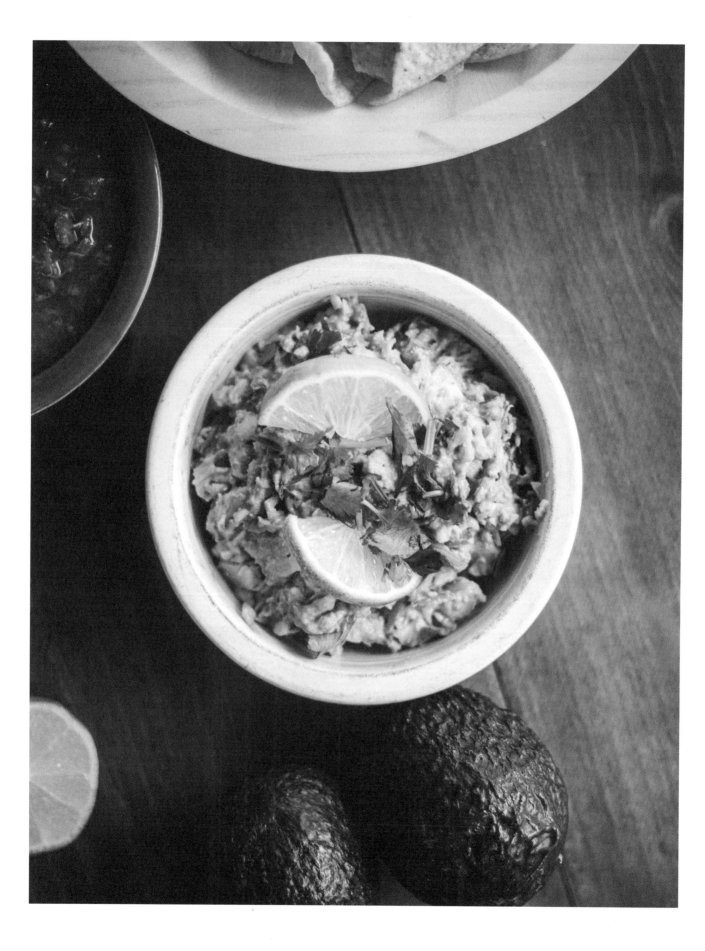

Guacamole

A party favorite, this guacamole mixes up in just minutes. Your choice of salsa will affect the guacamole's taste. We recommend making our fresh salsa with adjustable heat using jalapeño seeds. Good-quality jarred salsa can be substituted. Using a ripe avocado will make mashing easy and yield a creamy consistency. Serve as a dip for tortilla chips, or pair with any of your favorite recipes.

MAKES 1 CUP

2 avocados

2 cloves garlic, minced

¼ cup Fresh Salsa (p. 254)

juice of ½ lime

¼ teaspoon kosher salt

freshly ground black pepper

Mash the avocado using a fork. Stir in remaining ingredients, seasoning with pepper to taste.

USE IN THESE RECIPES

Breakfast Tacos (p. 46)

Seven-Layer Burrito Pan (p. 173)

Chorizo Quesadillas (p. 174)

Lemon Dill Spinach Artichoke Dip

Creamy, comforting, and chock-full of vegetables, this dip is much lower in fat and sodium than a restaurant appetizer version. Yet thanks to lemon and dill, it is full of bright flavor. This works well as a dip for vegetables or whole grain crackers or as a spread on bread or in sandwiches.

SERVES 12

8 ounces baby spinach or mature leaves, torn or chopped into pieces; or 10 ounces frozen, thawed and drained

1 (14-ounce) can artichoke hearts (plain, not marinated), drained; or 9 ounces freshly cooked or frozen, thawed and drained

8 ounces cream cheese, softened or Lebanese Labneh (p. 228)

1 cup Greek yogurt

2 green onions, chopped

2 cloves garlic, minced

¼ cup minced fresh dill weed; or 4 teaspoons dried

zest of 1 lemon

2-4 tablespoons freshly squeezed lemon juice

½ teaspoon kosher salt

¼ teaspoon freshly ground black pepper

GARNISHES

salt and pepper

Parmesan cheese

nutritional yeast

fresh dill weed

If using fresh spinach, wilt in a dry skillet over medium heat for about 2 minutes. If using thawed, previously frozen spinach, drain and squeeze out any extra water.

Place all ingredients, except garnishes, into a food processor. Pulse until well combined but not pureed.

Transfer mixture into an 8 x 8-inch baking pan or 2-quart baking dish. Place in a cold oven and turn to 350°F. Start timing and bake for 25 minutes, or until heated through and top is beginning to brown.

Sprinkle top with any or all garnishes if desired.

MAKE IT YOURSELF

Greek Yogurt (p. 280–281)

Poppy Seed Dressing

You can go two ways with this dressing. Make a traditional creamy version using plain Greek yogurt, or substitute oil for a clear vinaigrette.

MAKES ⅓ CUP

¼ cup plain Greek yogurt (for creamy) or canola oil (for clear)

1 tablespoon white wine or apple cider vinegar

2 teaspoons honey

1½ teaspoons poppy seeds

¼ teaspoon Dijon mustard

⅛ teaspoon kosher salt

½ teaspoon minced shallot (optional)

Whisk all dressing ingredients in a small bowl or shake them together in a jar with a tight-fitting lid.

USE IN THESE RECIPES

Summer Berry and Spinach Salad (p. 71)
Cruciferous Cranberry Crunch Salad (p. 76)

MAKE IT YOURSELF

Greek Yogurt (p. 280–281)

Vinaigrette

From dressing up greens to marinating beans, this simple dressing will infuse flavor into a variety of salads. Do-it-yourself dressings allow you to control salt and sweetness. Taste will be fresh, money will be saved, and packaging waste will be prevented! Use up any extra shallot in any recipe that calls for onion. Depending on the recipe, sometimes we call for a balsamic or red wine vinegar variation because of their distinct flavor characteristics.

MAKES ⅔ CUP

⅓ cup extra-virgin olive oil

2½ tablespoons balsamic or red wine vinegar

1½ tablespoons minced shallot

1½ teaspoons honey or maple syrup

1 teaspoon Dijon mustard

⅛ teaspoon kosher salt

⅛ teaspoon freshly ground black pepper

Whisk all dressing ingredients in a small bowl or shake them together in a jar with a tight-fitting lid.

USE IN THESE RECIPES

Pear Walnut Salad (p. 69)

Roasted Beet and Goat Cheese Salad (p. 70)

Summer Berry and Spinach Salad (p. 71)

Cruciferous Cranberry Crunch Salad (p. 76)

Balsamic Three Bean Salad (p. 86)

Avocado Dressing

Avocado lends its naturally creamy goodness to this dressing, which could complement many salads.

MAKES 1 CUP

---

1 ripe avocado

2 cloves garlic, minced

2 tablespoons extra-virgin olive oil

2 tablespoons lemon juice or apple cider vinegar

1 tablespoon Dijon mustard

¼ cup water plus additional to thin

¼ teaspoon kosher salt

freshly ground black pepper

2 tablespoons nutritional yeast (optional)

Combine all ingredients in a food processor or blender, adding pepper as desired. Process until smooth. You may add additional water 1 tablespoon at a time until the mixture reaches your desired dressing consistency. Be careful not to make it too watery, but you also want it to be pourable for dressing salad.

USE IN THESE RECIPES

Cobb Salad (p. 66)
Southwest Chopped Salad (p. 83)

Cilantro Lime Dressing

Some people have an aversion to cilantro, so in that case we suggest substituting parsley so as not to miss out on this delicious dressing.

MAKES ¾ CUP

½ cup chopped fresh cilantro or flat-leaf parsley

¼ cup extra-virgin olive oil

juice of 2 limes

2 teaspoons honey

1 teaspoon minced garlic

½ teaspoon chili powder

¼ teaspoon kosher salt

⅛ teaspoon freshly ground black pepper

1 small jalapeño, seeded and finely chopped (optional)

Whisk all dressing ingredients in a small bowl or shake them together in a jar with a tight-fitting lid.

USE IN THIS RECIPE

Southwest Chopped Salad (p. 83)

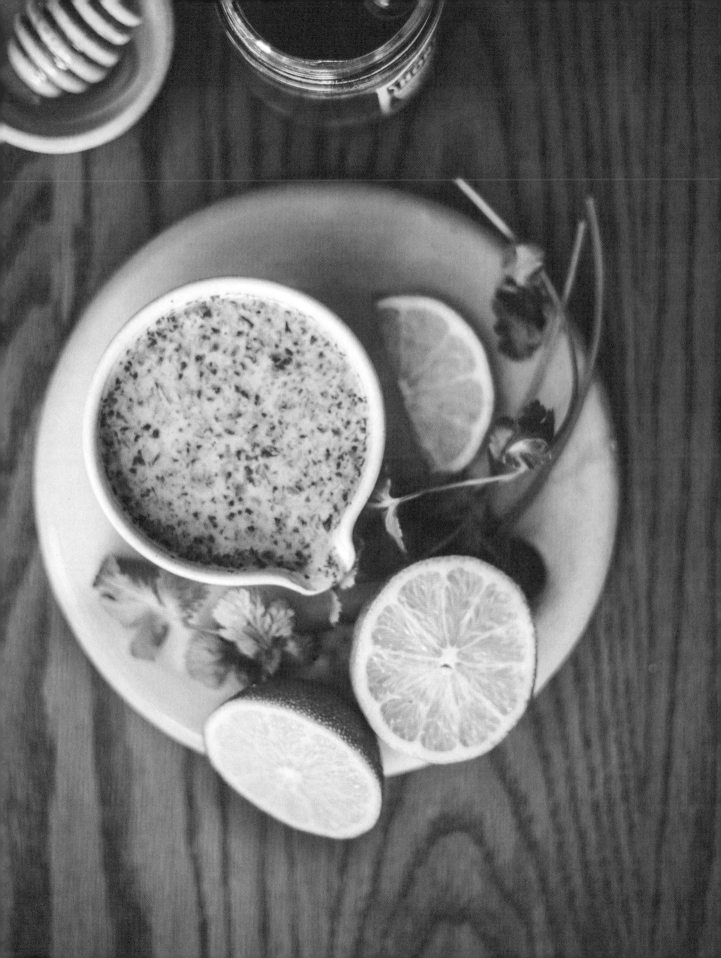

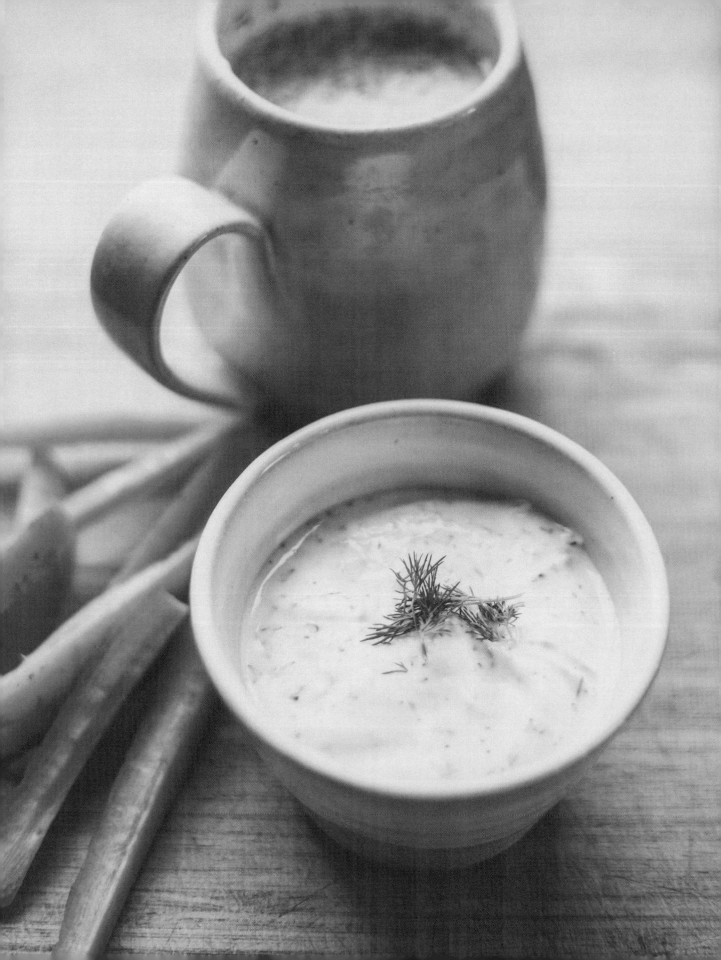

Ranch Dip or Buttermilk Ranch Dressing

So simple, this dip is made in under a minute! No ranch flavor packets, sour cream, or mayonnaise needed for this nutritious dip, which will make you want to eat your veggies. Thinning with buttermilk turns dip into a dressing.

MAKES 1 CUP DIP OR 1¼ CUPS DRESSING

RANCH DIP

1 cup plain Greek yogurt

½ teaspoon dried dill weed

½ teaspoon garlic powder

½ teaspoon onion powder

¼ teaspoon kosher salt

⅛ teaspoon freshly ground black pepper

BUTTERMILK RANCH DRESSING

All ingredients from Ranch Dip

⅓ cup buttermilk; or ¼ cup milk plus
1 teaspoon vinegar or lemon juice

In a small bowl, combine all the ingredients. Only add the buttermilk if you are making the dressing, as this will thin it enough to make it pourable. Stir and refrigerate.

MAKE IT YOURSELF

Greek Yogurt (p. 280–281)

Buttermilk (p. 282)

Lemon Garlic Tahini Dressing

This Greek- or Caesar-style dressing tastes great on a variety of salads.

MAKES ½ CUP

2 tablespoons tahini

2 tablespoons freshly squeezed lemon juice

2 tablespoons reduced sodium soy sauce or tamari

2 tablespoons apple cider vinegar

¼ cup nutritional yeast

2 teaspoons minced garlic

Whisk all dressing ingredients in a small bowl or shake them together in a jar with a tight-fitting lid.

USE IN THESE RECIPES

Zesty Garlic Kale Salad (p. 67)
Roasted Veggie and Chickpea Bowl (p. 150)

MAKE IT YOURSELF

Tahini (p. 273)

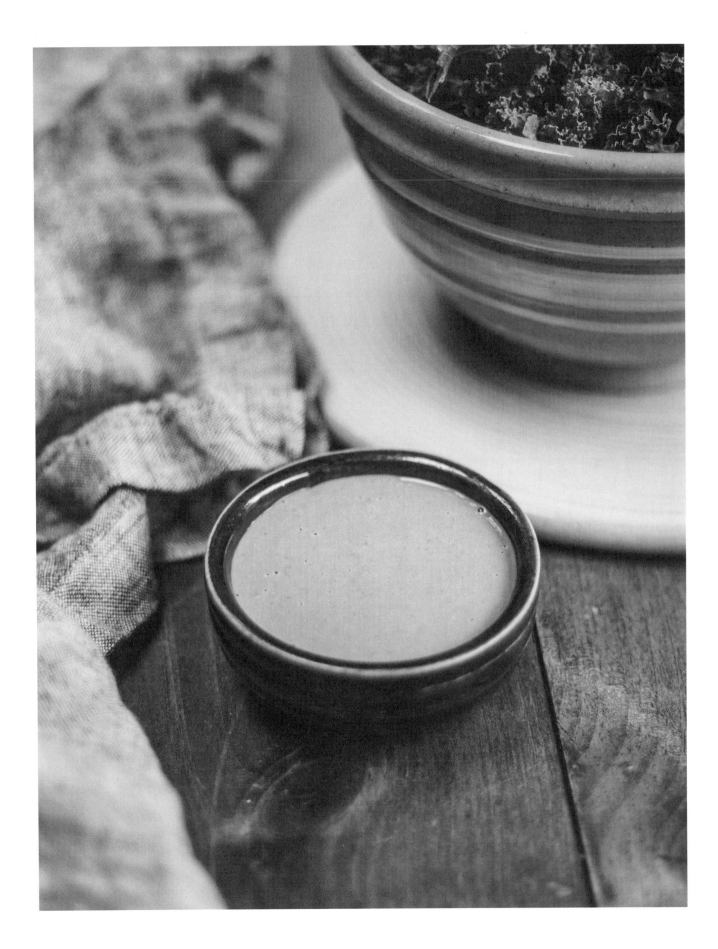

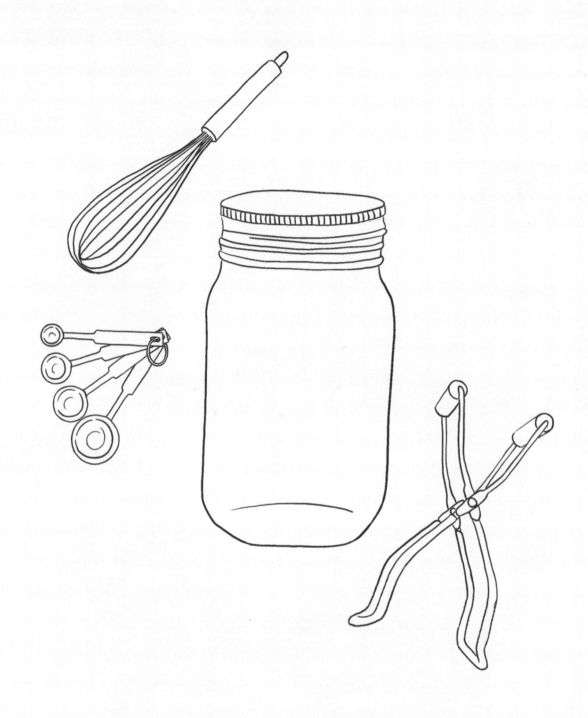

Make
It Yourself

———

Natural Nut or Seed Butters

If you have a food processor, you can make your own natural nut and seed butters in no time. We recommend making them unsweetened and unsalted but provide suggestions if you prefer sweet or salty. Nuts that work well include almonds, cashews, hazelnuts, peanuts, pecans, and pistachios; for seed butter, sunflower seeds work best.

MAKES 2 CUPS

4 cups unsalted nuts or seeds

1 teaspoon honey (optional)

½ teaspoon table salt (optional)

Spread nuts (or seeds) out on a baking sheet in a single layer. Place in a cold oven and turn to 375°F. Start timing. If starting with roasted nuts or seeds, warm in the oven for 10 minutes. If starting with raw nuts or seeds, roast for 15 minutes. Remove from oven and let cool for about 5 minutes.

Transfer nuts to the food processor. Process until desired consistency is achieved. Each variety of nut or seed will take a different amount of time to release its oil. Peanuts, pecans, hazelnuts, and shelled sunflower seeds are the quickest, at about 3 minutes. Cashews and pistachios take 5–10 minutes. Almonds take the longest—between 10 and 15 minutes. Stop often to scrape down sides of the bowl.

If desired, sweeten and season with our suggested amounts of honey and salt, then add more to taste. To thin, add a small amount of neutral-flavored oil, such as canola.

Refrigerate for up to 6 months.

USE IN THESE RECIPES

Energy Balls (p. 219)
Pumpkin Spice Dip (p. 225)
Peanut Sauce (p. 252)

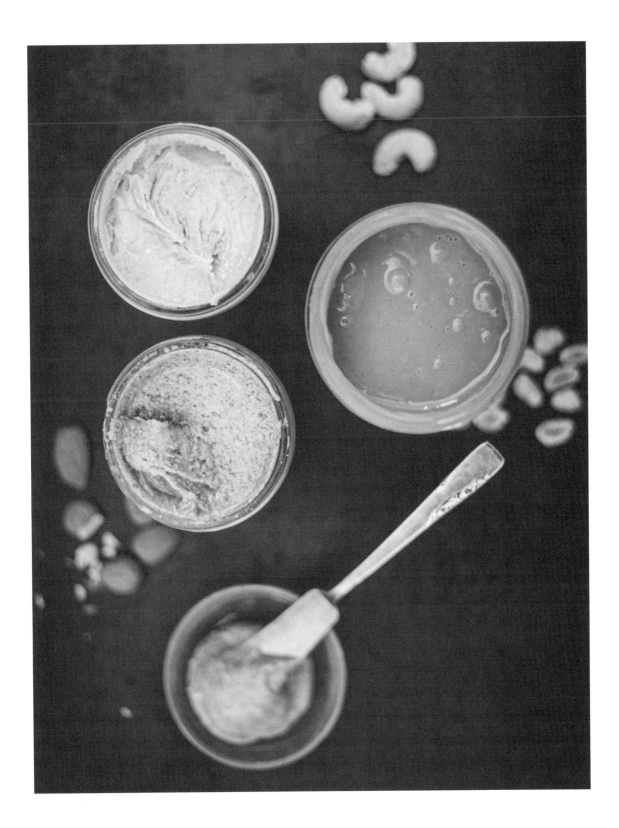

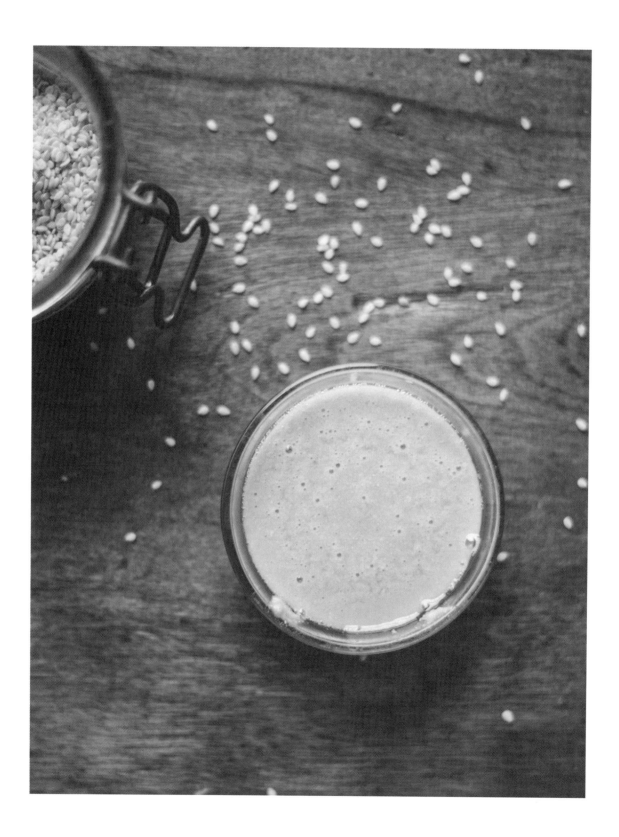

Tahini

Tahini, which is really just sesame seed butter, is made just as you would any nut or seed butter, with a touch of oil added in. Hulled white sesame seeds are what is most typically used, but any variety will work. If you can buy sesame seeds in bulk, homemade tahini will be much less expensive—and of course fresher—than store-bought tahini.

MAKES 1 CUP

---

2 cups sesame seeds

2-4 tablespoons canola oil

Toast sesame seeds (technique on p. 312).

Transfer toasted seeds to a food processor. Process about 2 minutes. Stop often to scrape down sides of the bowl. Add 2 tablespoons oil. Continue to process for another 1–2 minutes. If desired, thin with additional oil, adding about 1 tablespoon at a time until preferred consistency is achieved.

Refrigerate for up to 6 months.

USE IN THESE RECIPES

Classic Hummus (p. 251)
Lemon Garlic Tahini Dressing (p. 266)

Canned Diced Tomatoes

Canning fresh tomatoes in season captures fresh, local tomato taste that is better than anything you can buy. When a recipe calls for store-bought cans of tomato, know that a 14-ounce can is equivalent to 1 pint home-canned tomatoes, and a 28-ounce can is equal to 1 homemade quart.

YIELDS VARY

FOR EACH QUART JAR:

about 3 pounds tomatoes

2 tablespoons lemon juice

1 teaspoon kosher salt (optional)

Prepare everything needed for canning according to the boiling-water method (technique on p. 305).

Determine how many tomatoes you plan to can and whether you want to can quarts, pints, or a mix. If you want some pints of tomatoes, use half the ingredients on the list above per pint. Then determine how many jars you need.

Prepare tomatoes: Blanch tomatoes to remove skins (you can leave skins on; however, they get tough during canning). Fill a clean sink, cooler, or very large bowl with ice water. Bring a large pot of water to boil. Use a knife to score an X on the bottom of each tomato. Place several tomatoes at a time in the boiling water and blanch until the skins begin to loosen, 45–60 seconds. Scoop out tomatoes with a slotted spoon and plunge them into the ice water to stop the cooking. Continue blanching in batches until all tomatoes are done. Remove tomatoes from the cold water and slip off their skins; then core them with a paring knife. Dice them into any size that you desire. Compost skins.

Put lemon juice and optional salt into each of the clean, hot jars. Fill jars with tomatoes, pressing them in gently but firmly to release air pockets and letting juice come over the top of the tomatoes. Leave ½ inch headspace between the surface of the tomato juice and the top of the jar. Release any air pockets or bubbles by running a bubble tool or chopstick around the inside edge of the jar.

Proceed with canning using the boiling-water method, picking back up where you left off in the canning technique on page 306. Canner processing time for tomatoes is 85 minutes; adjust time as needed for higher elevations.

USE IN THESE RECIPES

Any of the many in this cookbook that call for canned tomatoes!

Roasted Red Peppers

These are easy to make: simply put the pepper very close to high heat, charring its outer skin while roasting it underneath.

MAKES ¾ CUP (EQUIVALENT TO A 7-OUNCE STORE-BOUGHT JAR)

2 medium red bell peppers

Roast bell peppers using either an oven broiler or a gas range stovetop:

Broiling method: Core, seed, and quarter bell peppers. Place skin side up on a baking sheet. Broil 5–10 minutes until the pepper skins turn black.

Gas range method: Place whole bell peppers directly on the stovetop grates over an open flame, medium heat. Use tongs to rotate the peppers several times each minute, charring their skins, which will blacken and blister, 5–10 minutes.

Place roasted peppers in a bowl and cover tightly. Let cool 10–15 minutes. Gently peel away and compost the skins. If you used the stovetop method, cut away the stems and remove the seeds.

USE IN THESE RECIPES

Antipasto Platter or Sandwich (p. 119)

Portabella Mushroom Burgers (p. 127)

Spring Veggie and Pesto Pasta (p. 137)

Classic Hummus, roasted red pepper variation (p. 251)

Whole Wheat Tortillas, roasted red pepper wrap variation (p. 286–287)

Dilly Beans

Dill weed and dill seed lend double dilly-delicious flavor to these green beans, which are a nice alternative to the more traditional cucumber dill pickle. Open a jar and it'll soon be gone—especially if there are kids in the house.

MAKES 7 PINT JARS

---

3 pounds green beans, tops trimmed

5 cups distilled white vinegar

2½ cups water

¼ cup honey

2½ tablespoons kosher salt

7 cloves garlic, sliced thin

1 cup fresh dill weed

2 tablespoons dill seed

1 tablespoon black peppercorns

Make preparations for canning using the boiling-water method (technique on p. 305).

Trim green beans to about 3¼ inches in length. You will want them to be about 1 inch below the top of a pint jar when packed in vertically. Save shorter trimmings, as these can also be used by packing and stacking in and around each other to fill in jar space if needed.

Prepare the brine: In a medium saucepan, combine vinegar, water, honey, and salt. Bring to a boil, then reduce heat to low to keep hot until ready for use.

Pack beans into the hot canning jars fairly tightly but with enough room for adding the herbs and spices. In each jar, add some garlic slices, dill weed, dill seed, and peppercorns so that these ingredients are distributed relatively evenly between the jars.

Set the canning funnel on a jar and ladle in hot brine, covering the beans by about ½ inch and leaving about ½ inch headspace (space between the surface of the liquid and the top of the jar). Release any air pockets or bubbles by running a bubble tool or chopstick around the inside edge of the jar.

Proceed with canning using the boiling-water method, picking back up where you left off in the technique on page 306. Canner processing time for dilly beans is 15 minutes; adjust time as needed for higher elevations.

USE IN THIS RECIPE

Crunchy Hummus Veggie Wrap (p. 123)

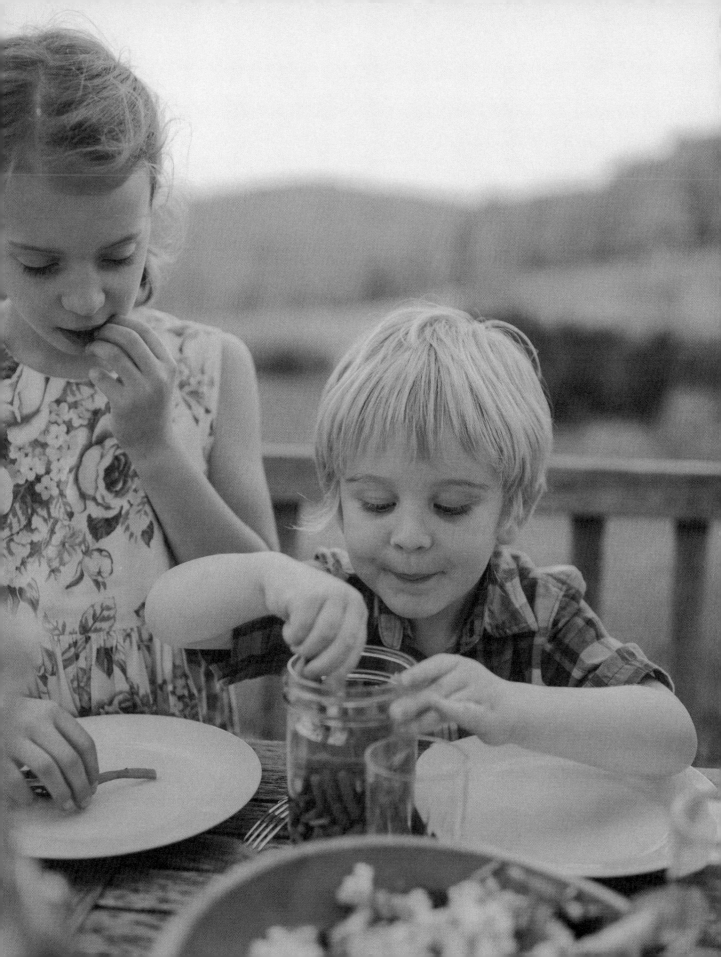

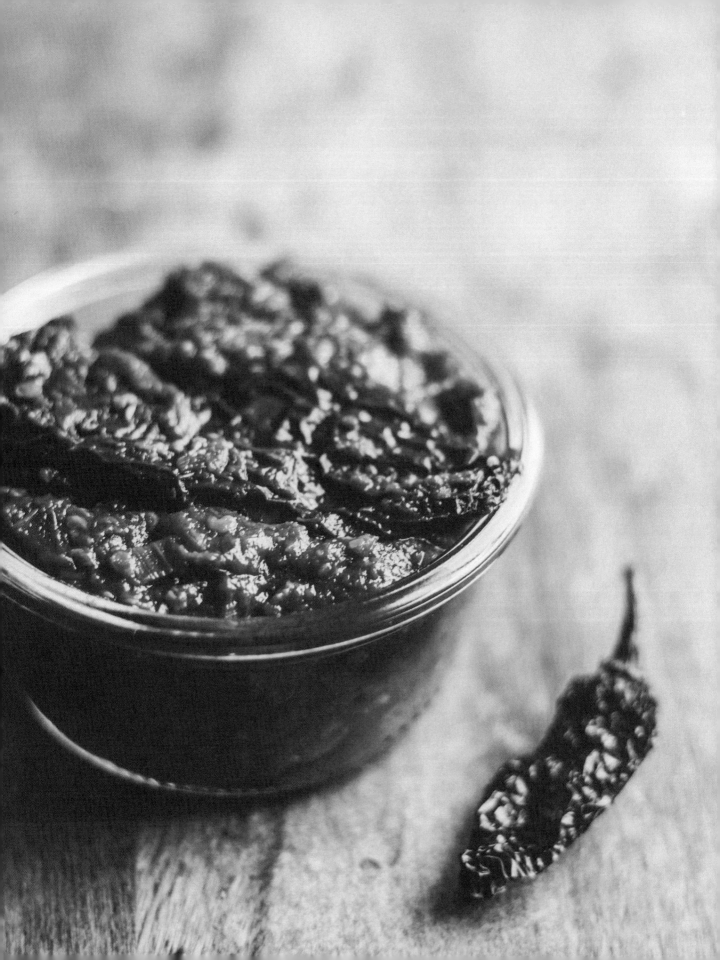

Chipotle Peppers in Adobo Sauce

If you have access to dried chipotle peppers (smoked jalapeños), make your own canned chipotle peppers in adobo sauce and save a can. Dried chipotle peppers can be found in grocery stores near bulk spices or with Mexican items in international food sections. Freeze extra prepared peppers individually with a bit of sauce in ice cube trays and then put into freezer bags for later use.

MAKES 8 CHIPOTLE PEPPERS IN 1 CUP ADOBO SAUCE

12 dried chipotle peppers, stems removed

2 cups water

¾ cup tomato puree or canned tomatoes

½ teaspoon honey (optional)

1 onion, chopped

4 cloves garlic, minced

⅓ cup apple cider vinegar

½ teaspoon ground cumin

½ teaspoon kosher salt

Place chipotle peppers in a saucepan with water. Bring to a boil. Turn off heat. Submerge the peppers in the hot water by placing a small plate or lid directly on the water's surface. Let peppers soak for about 20 minutes. Leave 8 peppers in the water. Remove 4 and put them into a blender or food processor with tomato puree and optional honey, if desired. Puree until smooth.

Add puree back into the saucepan with the 8 peppers and soaking water. Add all remaining ingredients: onion, garlic, vinegar, cumin, and salt. Bring to a simmer, partly cover, and cook over low heat for about 1 hour, or until reduced to about 1 cup. Peek in the saucepan from time to time and stir, making sure there is still sufficient liquid to prevent burning.

USE IN THESE RECIPES

Chipotle Pumpkin Chili (p. 101)
Cauliflower Tacos (p. 170)
Spicy Cauliflower Walnut Chorizo (p. 197)

Yogurt or Greek Yogurt

Making yogurt is easy. Even though it takes a while, it requires very little active cooking time. Homemade yogurt will save you money and reduce plastic waste, especially if you have the option of buying milk in glass bottles. Whole milk makes the thickest yogurt, but any fat level will work. For your first batch of yogurt, you can use store-bought plain yogurt as the starter culture; for future batches, use your own homemade yogurt.

MAKES 4 CUPS REGULAR OR 2 CUPS GREEK

---

4 cups (1 quart) fresh milk

¼ cup plain yogurt containing live, active cultures

The plain yogurt needs to be at room temperature. Measure out ¼ cup yogurt and let stand at room temperature while you heat and cool your milk. (If you forget to bring the yogurt to room temperature, you can temper it: warm cold yogurt by whisking in a bit of the heated and cooled milk when you get to that step.)

Heat milk to just under a boil, about 190°F. You'll start to see the surface of the milk moving and tiny bubbles beginning to form. This heating step kills any bacteria in the milk. Remove from heat and let milk cool down to about 110°F, or until you can comfortably put a clean pinkie finger into it for 10 seconds or so. This cooling step is important so as not to kill the good bacteria, which will be added next. (You can expedite the cooling process by setting the pot of milk in a bowl of ice water.)

Skim off any skin that has formed on the milk's surface. Whisk the room-temperature or tempered plain yogurt into the cooled but still-warm milk. This step adds the culture-containing probiotics, which will transform your milk into yogurt.

Pour the mixture into a heatproof container. A glass quart jar works well. A funnel can be helpful for easy pouring. Put a lid on the jar after filling.

Now the yogurt needs to sit, undisturbed, in a warm spot for at least 6 hours. A corner of the kitchen counter is ideal. The amount of time it takes the yogurt to set will depend on the surrounding temperature. Keeping the yogurt at a consistently warm temperature is the goal. About 110°F is an ideal temperature for fermentation to happen. There are different ways to do this. You can wrap kitchen towels or blankets around the jar; put the mixture in a thermos to help regulate the temperature; place in a prewarmed oven with the light on but heat off; or wrap in a heating pad. A yogurt maker works as well.

After about 6 hours, check to see if yogurt has set by tilting the jar and noting if the top has solidified. If not yet set and still too liquid, leave the jar and check again in another 1 or 2 hours.

Once yogurt is set, refrigerate until cold, about 2 hours. After it is chilled, you can make Greek yogurt (see below) if you'd like. Store for up to 1 week.

Make sure to save some yogurt so that you

can start your next batch. Measuring out ¼ cup from your fresh batch of yogurt right away and putting it aside in a small container will ensure you've always got your next starter culture when you need it.

GREEK YOGURT

Makes 2 cups

Greek yogurt, also known as yogurt cheese, is simply yogurt that has been drained to remove some of the liquid whey. This makes it thicker.

4 cups (1 quart) regular plain yogurt

Make yogurt as above, or purchase a quart of plain yogurt. Suspend a colander or fine-mesh sieve over a bowl and line the colander with several layers of cheesecloth. After the yogurt has been chilled, spoon it into the middle of the colander. Cover and refrigerate for several hours or up to a full day, depending on thickness desired. After draining, scoop Greek yogurt back into a container for storage.

The liquid whey is a protein by-product from making Greek yogurt. It is considered sweet whey (as opposed to the acid whey by-product from cheese making). This whey can be used as a substitute for buttermilk or to replace some or all the liquid in any bread recipe. Try it in our Whole Grain Pancakes (p. 53–54) or Honey-Oat Breakfast Bread (p. 59). You can use it for cooking grains (oatmeal, rice, pasta) or add it to soup or smoothies. If you won't use it up within 1 week, freeze whey for later use.

USE IN THESE RECIPES

Any of the many in this cookbook that call for yogurt!

Butter and Buttermilk

Fresh cream + food processor + five minutes = butter. You can also hand shake cream into butter in 15 minutes using a quart jar with tight fitting lid. What a simple equation! Seeing as cream is the only ingredient needed, the quality of the cream matters. If available, choose local, fresh cream without any additives. To make flavored herb butter (also known as compound butter), simply add herbs.

MAKES 6-8 OUNCES BUTTER (ABOUT 16 TABLESPOONS) PLUS 1 CUP BUTTERMILK

2 cups (1 pint) whipping or heavy cream

salt (optional)

Pour cream into a food processor. Turn on and begin to process. The S-blade will begin to churn the cream, first into whipped cream, and then continuing into butter.

You'll know you've got butter when the whipped cream collapses, turns grainy in texture, yellow in color, and releases its liquid (the buttermilk). As soon as you see or hear the buttermilk liquid separating from the butter, turn off the food processor.

Use a fine-mesh sieve to drain off the buttermilk, saving it to use with other recipes (see below).

With the butter still in the sieve, run it under cold water until the rinse water becomes clear and is no longer cloudy. Put the butter in a small bowl. Use a spatula to press the butter against the side of the bowl, squeezing out and draining off all liquid. Buttermilk that is not removed will cause the butter to spoil.

USE BUTTERMILK IN THESE RECIPES

Whole Grain Pancakes or Waffles (p. 53–54)
Buttermilk Ranch Dressing (p. 265)

Mix in salt, if desired. Unsalted is recommended if you are using the butter for baking and also works well in cooking since you will be adding salt to taste. If you want to make a regular salted equivalent to store-bought butter, add ½ teaspoon salt. You could also mix in less for a lower-sodium butter. Serve soft or refrigerate to harden and store for up to 3 weeks.

ADDITIONAL INGREDIENTS FOR COMPOUND BUTTER VARIATION

finely chopped fresh herbs such as parsley, sage, rosemary, thyme, dill, cilantro, chive, basil, or a combination

other flavors, such as minced garlic or shallot, a squeeze of lemon or lime juice, a drizzle of extra-virgin olive oil, a crack of fresh pepper, or a dash of paprika

The ratio of butter to herbs can be to taste. A typical ratio is 1 tablespoon finely chopped fresh herbs mixed into 4 ounces freshly made soft butter; however, you can use more or less to taste. Have fun and experiment with adding other flavors.

USE BUTTER IN THESE RECIPES

Honey-Oat Breakfast Bread (p. 59)
Caprese Grilled Cheese (p. 118)
Root Vegetable Potpie (p. 131)
Lentil Shepherd's Pie (p. 134)
Foraged Fiddleheads (p. 185)
Honey Roasted Peanuts (p. 214–215)
Cran-Apple Crisp (p. 226)

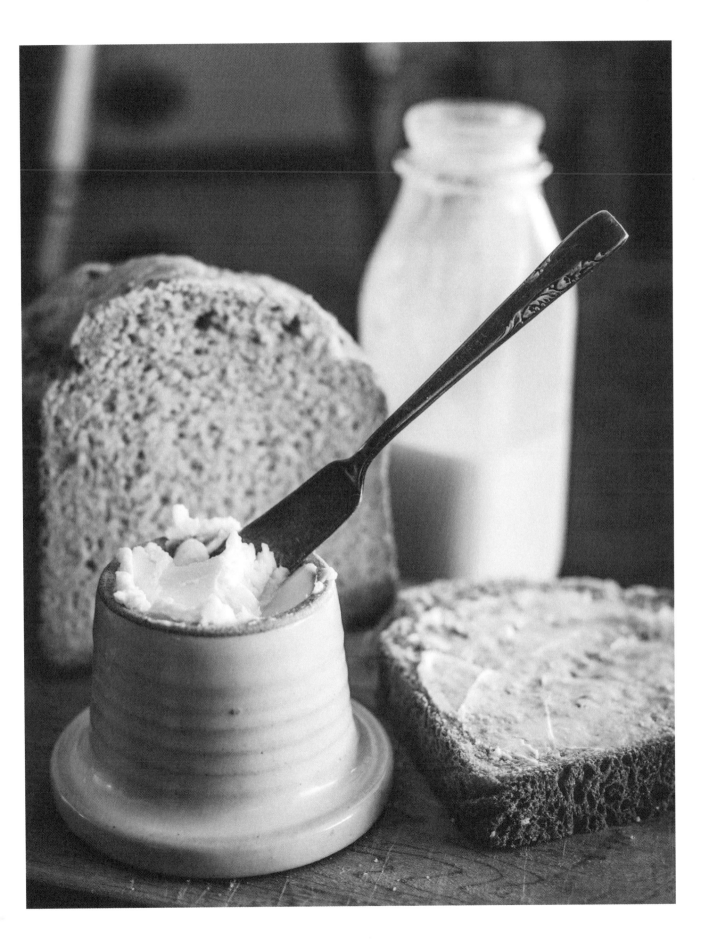

QUALITY TIME

Confession: most of my free time is spent in the kitchen, the garden, and the grocery store. Yet I wouldn't have it any other way. Feeding our family in this manner is a top priority for me, and even though it consumes my time, it gives me life. And it is quality time. We eat all our meals at home together as a family, giving thanks for our food, touching base on the day before us at breakfast and recounting our days over dinner at the dining room table. While my husband washes dishes and I put away leftovers and pack lunches, we get to continue our conversations at a deeper level.

Often, when I am working outside, my girls are by my side: planting seeds, picking potato bugs, collecting the eggs. When I am in the kitchen, they are mixing ingredients, setting the table, or emptying the compost pail. In doing these things, they are being exposed to nature, gaining practical skills, growing in confidence, developing a work ethic, and feeling a sense of purpose.

My hope is that our lifestyle and life lessons learned now will lead to a legacy of resilience. Challenges will inevitably unfold during my children's lifetime, and we pray that the quality time we've invested today will be rendered into good memories and helpful skills.

Mayonnaise

Easily made in a food processor with small bowl attachment or using immersion blender, mayonnaise can also be whisked by hand. Mayonnaise is made with raw egg, so this recipe is not recommended for anyone with a compromised immune system.

MAKES ½ CUP

1 egg, at room temperature

1 tablespoon lemon juice;
or ½ tablespoon vinegar + ½ tablespoon water

¼ teaspoon dry mustard

¼ teaspoon salt

dash freshly ground black pepper, cayenne, or a combination (optional)

½ cup canola oil

USE IN THIS RECIPE

Chipotle Mayo (p.170)

In a small bowl, combine egg, lemon juice, dry mustard, salt, and optional pepper, if desired. Mayonnaise can be emulsified by hand whisking, with an immersion blender, or in a small bowl attachment of a food processor with the center piece in the lid removed to allow you to add in oil. Begin to whisk, blend, or process. Very slowly, start adding the oil in a very thin stream or even drop by drop. This slow pace is key to emulsification. The mixture will thicken up and lighten in color as it begins to emulsify. Once this occurs, you may stream in any remaining oil at a slightly faster flow.

Store in the refrigerator for up to 1 week.

Note: For fail-proof mayo that thickens and doesn't break its emulsion, use room temperature ingredients, use a small bowl so mixture has enough contact with the blade or whisk (otherwise you may end up with mayo soup), add in oil very, very slowly so each fat droplet can become emulsified into the mixture.

Whole Wheat Tortillas

Making your own tortillas is fun, and they taste much fresher than anything you can buy. If you can't find spelt, an ancient, sweet-tasting wheat variety, substitute with white whole wheat flour or try the corn variation. No matter what grain combination you use, these are 100 percent whole grain. Spinach and roasted red pepper wrap variations are also included here.

MAKES 8 (7-INCH) TORTILLAS

1½ cups (190 grams) whole wheat flour or white whole wheat

1 cup (117 grams) whole spelt flour or white whole wheat (127 grams)

¾ teaspoon kosher salt

¾ cup plus 2 tablespoons water

¼ cup olive or avocado oil

In a medium bowl, whisk together both flours and salt.

Add water and oil. Stir until dough comes together into a ball. Turn ball of dough out onto a floured surface. Knead until smooth. Put dough back into the bowl and cover with a clean kitchen towel. Let rest for about 15 minutes.

Divide dough into eight equal pieces, about 2½ ounces each. Using your hands, flatten each ball slightly into a round disc. Working with one piece at a time, roll a disc of dough into an 8-inch circle (it will end up shrinking by an inch or so). If you have a tortilla press, it makes easy work of this; otherwise a rolling pin works just fine. (A trick to keeping tortillas from sticking to surfaces: Take a gallon-sized resealable bag. Zip up the top. Cut the seams on all three other sides. Center the ball of dough between the two plastic sheets. Now you can roll or press the dough without it sticking to your rolling pin, the counter, or your press. Save this bag to reuse next time you make tortillas.)

Heat a skillet or griddle over medium heat. Cast iron, if you have it, is a great choice. Once hot, add the tortilla you've just rolled. Cook no more than 1 minute, then flip and cook on the other side for about 30 seconds. You want the tortilla to bubble and brown slightly but remain soft so that it will be flexible. After you've cooked one tortilla, press and cook the next tortilla, repeating the sequence until all eight have been pressed and cooked.

Corn variation: Replace the 1 cup spelt flour with 1 cup (105 grams) masa harina corn flour. Increase water to 1 cup.

Spinach variation: Substitute spinach puree for the water: Measure out 1 cup spinach (either sautéed or 10 ounces frozen spinach, thawed and drained). Puree this, then pour into a liquid measuring cup. If needed, add enough water to constitute the ¾ cup plus 2 tablespoons liquid volume needed. Use this in the recipe when water is called for.

Roasted red pepper variation: Substitute roasted red pepper puree for the ¾ cup water: Measure out ¾ cup roasted red peppers that have been drained from their jar; or make your own (p. 275). Puree this, then pour into a liquid measuring cup. Add enough water to constitute the ¾ cup plus 2 tablespoons liquid volume needed.

Use this in the recipe when water is called for.

USE IN THESE RECIPES

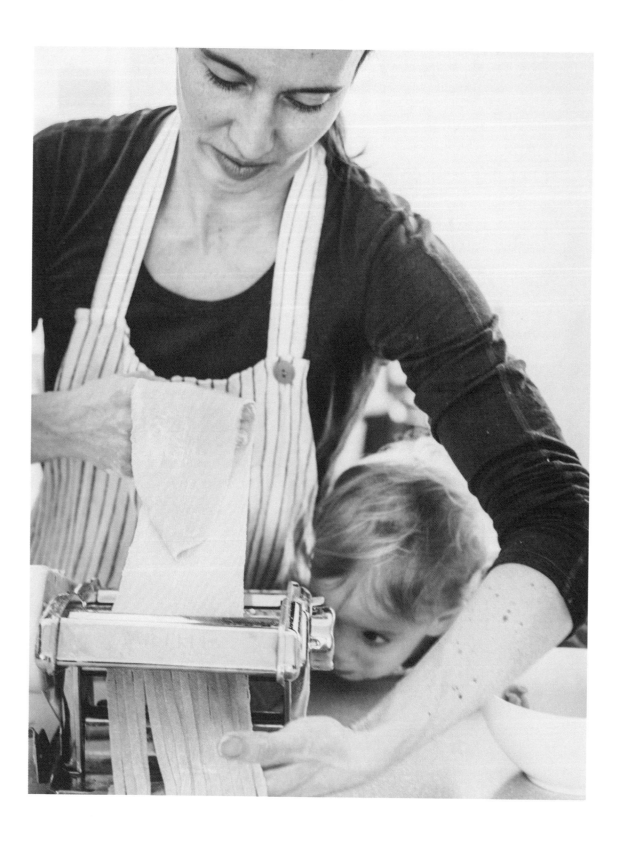

Fresh Pasta

Homemade egg pasta is worth making and can be done entirely by hand or aided by machine. This recipe calls for an equal blend of two flours; however, you can use all white or go 100 percent whole wheat if you prefer. Tastes better than boxed pasta, and it saves a box too.

MAKES 12 OUNCES (SERVES 6)

---

1 cup (127 grams) white whole wheat flour

1 cup (123 grams) all-purpose flour

3 eggs

½ teaspoon table salt

½–1 tablespoon extra-virgin olive oil (optional)

Measure the flours (technique on p. 310–311).

You can make pasta dough by hand, using a food processor, or a mixer with a dough hook.

By hand: Pour flour into a pile on the counter. Create a well in the middle of the flour and pour eggs, salt, and optional oil inside. Use a fork to whisk the eggs, then start incorporating the flour to achieve a wet, sticky dough. A bench scraper is nice to help you work with the dough. Knead dough until smooth and elastic.

By food processor: Add all the ingredients and pulse until combined and crumbly, then turn on and process continuously until dough starts to come together, about 1 minute. Stop to scrape down the sides as needed. Remove dough and knead several times until it comes together in a smooth, elastic ball.

By mixer: Add all ingredients to the mixer bowl with the eggs in the center. Use a fork to first whisk the eggs and then incorporate the flour until everything is combined. Use the dough hook attachment and mix until dough is smooth and elastic, about 5 minutes.

After dough is mixed, shape into a ball and place in a clean bowl. Cover and refrigerate for 30 minutes.

(continued next page)

Divide dough into four pieces. Work with one at a time, keeping the others covered. Shape dough into a thick disc, then roll it out, using either a pasta maker according to the manufacturer's instructions or a rolling pin by hand. For hand rolling, keep counter and dough surfaces dusted with flour to prevent dough from sticking.

Moving the dough often during rolling also helps, reflouring as needed. Roll the stiff dough into a rectangular sheet as thin as possible. Then cut into the noodle shape that you desire—either with a pasta machine or a sharp chef's knife. Dust cut noodles with flour to prevent them from sticking to each other. Loosely fold them into small nests. If not cooking within 2 hours, store in an airtight container and refrigerate for up to 2 days.

Depending on thickness, fresh pasta usually takes 2–4 minutes, after placing in boiling water, to cook al dente.

For later use, fresh pasta can also be frozen flat on a baking sheet and then transferred to an airtight container stored in the freezer for up to 3 months. Frozen pasta will cook in 3–5 minutes, depending on size. Pasta can also be dried by laying it flat on a baking sheet, uncovered, for 12–24 hours. Turn pasta several times. Pasta can also be hung over clothes hangers or clothes drying racks until dry and brittle. Dried pasta can be stored in an airtight container for several weeks. Air dried pasta will cook in 4-6 minutes, depending on its size.

USE IN THESE RECIPES

Veggie Layered Lasagna (p. 140)
Pumpkin Parmesan Sage Pasta (p. 138)
Spring Veggie and Pesto Pasta (p. 137)
Hearty White Bean Ratatouille (p. 151)

Whole Wheat Bread Crumbs or Croutons

Make your own plain or seasoned bread crumbs or croutons from scraps of bread. Heels, crusts, stale slices: you can save all such scraps in your freezer and thaw out when ready to make a batch. Seasonings that work well include dried herbs, garlic powder, onion powder, kosher salt, and freshly ground black pepper.

YIELDS VARY

leftover whole wheat bread

seasonings (see headnote)

FOR CROUTONS

olive oil, butter, or a combination

USE BREAD CRUMBS IN THIS RECIPE

Crispy Tofu Parmesan with Sautéed Mushrooms (p. 132)

USE CROUTONS IN THIS RECIPE

Eat Your "Weeds" Salad (p. 72)

Thaw any bread that has been previously frozen.

Create a seasoning mix, if desired. Mix together any combination of dried herbs (an Italian mix is nice), garlic powder, onion powder, salt, and pepper. You will need about 1 teaspoon seasoning per 1 cup bread crumbs or cubes.

Bread crumbs: Put any amount of bread you've collected into a food processor. Process until desired crumb size, ranging from coarse to fine, is achieved.

Spread out crumbs in a single layer on a baking sheet. Let dry at room temperature for a day—the top of the refrigerator is a good, out-of-the-way place—or expedite drying by toasting in a 350°F oven for 10–15 minutes. No need to preheat. Mix in seasonings. Cool completely before storing. Store in the freezer for up to 1 year.

Croutons: Slice bread into bite-sized pieces. Place oil or butter in a skillet over medium heat, about 1 tablespoon per cup of cubed bread. Add bread pieces. Stir until beginning to brown. Remove from heat. Stir in seasonings while croutons are still in the hot skillet. Cool completely before storing—up to 1 week at room temperature or longer in the freezer.

KIDS IN THE KITCHEN

Cooking in our house is not always a meditative experience. As much as I love it when it is, I also love when my enthusiastic, eager-to-learn kids join me in the kitchen. Most parents can agree, sometimes they are hangry, eager-to-distract kids, but they are doing their important, age-appropriate job of learning about everything and everyone. Jacob, three years old, is very interested in cooking. He wishes he could do it all, but I let him do safe tasks like add the ingredients I've measured, stirring, and tearing broccoli and cauliflower florets into bite-sized pieces. Silas, nine months old, is the human vacuum under our feet, occasionally crying to be held because he likes to get a better look at what all those noises are and to see what he can taste. Cooking with kids can feel like a circus, but the more consistent we are about cooking together, the quicker they learn—both that parents can't always give them undivided attention and that they can help.

Vegetable Broth

Homemade broth is simple. Making your own will save packaging waste and allow you to control the amount of salt. This recipe is easily doubled, as any extra freezes well. You can save vegetable scraps in your freezer until you have enough.

MAKES 4 CUPS (1 QUART)

---

8 cups water

1 onion, quartered (with skin if desired)

2 ribs celery, roughly chopped

3 carrots, roughly chopped

3 cloves garlic, peeled and crushed using side of a knife blade

4 sprigs parsley, or ¼ teaspoon dried

4 sprigs thyme, or ¼ teaspoon dried

1 bay leaf

1 teaspoon whole peppercorns

up to 1 teaspoon kosher salt

6 mushrooms, halved (optional)

1 small potato, quartered (optional)

1 corn cob (optional)

1 leek, roughly chopped (optional)

Place all ingredients in a large saucepan or soup pot. For regular broth, use 1 teaspoon salt; for reduced sodium, use ½ teaspoon; for low sodium, use ¼ teaspoon; or omit salt entirely.

Bring to a boil. Reduce heat and simmer on low, partly covered, for 1 hour. Strain broth, pouring through a fine-mesh sieve. Eat any of the boiled vegetables that appeal to you. Compost the remaining solids. Broth is now ready to use immediately or be stored. Once cool, broth can be transferred to airtight containers and stored in the refrigerator for up to 1 week or in the freezer for up to 3 months.

USE IN THESE RECIPES

Any of the many in this cookbook that call for vegetable broth!

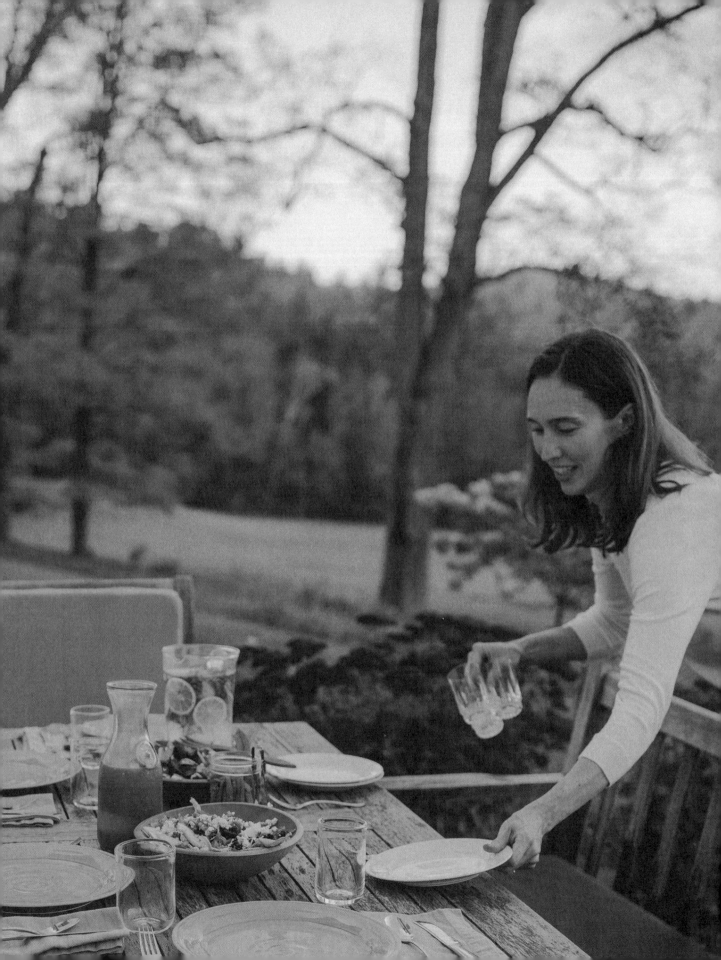

Meal Planning

One of the most important strategies to eating healthy and preventing food waste is to have a meal plan. It also helps you save money and decreases the last-minute stress of wondering what to make for dinner. Here are some general meal planning and prep tips.

START WITH WHAT YOU HAVE ON HAND. Are there items in your freezer, fridge, and pantry that need to be used? Be sure to incorporate those foods into the plan.

USE MYPLATE AS A GUIDE. Aim to make a meal that fills half the plate with colorful fruits or vegetables, one-quarter with grains (whole grains at least half the time), and one-quarter with protein.[4]

SNACKS SHOULD BE NUTRITIOUS. See snacks as opportunities to help you get all your food groups in during the course of the day. A combination of fiber and protein is satiating and a great choice to avoid overeating.

PLAN FOR LEFTOVERS. Work leftovers into your meal plan several times throughout the week to use things up. Have some frozen soups, stews, or chilis on hand in case you eat through your fresh foods faster than planned.

VARY YOUR VEGGIES. When you are making your meal plan, think about "eating the rainbow." Consider what colors you will consume, aiming to get a variety from all five subgroupings: reds/oranges, dark greens, starchy, legumes, and other (such as mushrooms and onions).

PLAN TO COOK ONE RECIPE AND USE IT SEVERAL WAYS. In the sample meal plan on the next page, the cilantro lime slaw is used in both wraps and tacos; hummus is used as a snack dip and sandwich spread; guacamole can go with the burrito recipe and as a snack dip with chips.

PLAN TO USE UP FRESH INGREDIENTS. In the sample meal plan, plain yogurt is used for granola, in the ranch dip, and for the smoothie. Kale is called for in both the roasted veggie and chickpea bowl and the kale chips.

PLAN SO THAT STURDIER INGREDIENTS APPEAR AT THE END OF THE WEEK and more perishable produce gets used up first, closer to when you've shopped. Salads and raw veggies are front-loaded toward the beginning, while root vegetable recipes come later.

PLAN TO USE YOUR RESOURCES EFFICIENTLY. Use your time well: Chop up all the raw veggies you plan to use over the next few days—for example, red bell pepper and cucumber strips to go in the wraps, more red bell pepper and carrots for the veggie bowl, some extras of everything to dip in hummus and ranch for snacks. Mix up dressings in advance so recipes come together quicker. You can prep the balsamic vinaigrette, peanut sauce, cilantro lime dressing, and pesto ahead of time. Use your oven well: Roast all your veggies for the week at the same time, while the oven is hot. In the sample meal plan below, you could cook three baking sheets at once: beets (for the salad), cauliflower (for the tacos), and sweet potato and chickpeas (for the veggie bowl). Note: Even though our recipe for roasting beets is written at a higher temp (450°F) than the cauliflower and sweet potato recipes, you can put them all in at 400°F and just leave the beets in longer than called for. With cooking you can take liberties. You are empowered and encouraged to experiment! Use your freezer well: Many recipes are freezer-friendly and make for healthy, quick options when you need a fast meal or one without much prep. Make ahead and freeze when you have time or when foods are in peak season.

day one	Breakfast	Honey-Oat Breakfast Bread with Natural Nut Butter, Pear
	Snack	Classic Hummus with veggies
	Lunch	Thai Veggie Tofu Wrap with Peanut Sauce and Cilantro Lime Slaw
	Snack	1 cup soup (any kind)
	Dinner	Seven-Layer Burrito Pan

day two	Breakfast	Simple Granola, Yogurt, Berries
	Snack	Energy Ball
	Lunch	Pita with Hummus, Roasted Beet and Goat Cheese Salad
	Snack	Edamame Caprese Salad
	Dinner	Leftover Seven-Layer Burrito Pan

day three	Breakfast	Veggie-Studded Frittata, Clementine
	Snack	Baked Blueberry Oatmeal Bites
	Lunch	Cauliflower Tacos with Cilantro Lime Slaw
	Snack	Spiced nuts, Grapes or raisins
	Dinner	Roasted Veggie and Chickpea Bowl

day four	Breakfast	Maple Walnut French Toast (using leftover Honey-Oat Breakfast Bread)
	Snack	Applesauce, Simple Granola
	Lunch	Lentil Shepherd's Pie
	Snack	Ranch Dip with veggies
	Dinner	Leftovers

day five	Breakfast	Berry Banana Smoothie
	Snack	Morning Glory Muffin
	Lunch	Sweet Potato Chili, Kale Chips
	Snack	Guacamole and Fresh Salsa with tortilla chips
	Dinner	Leftovers

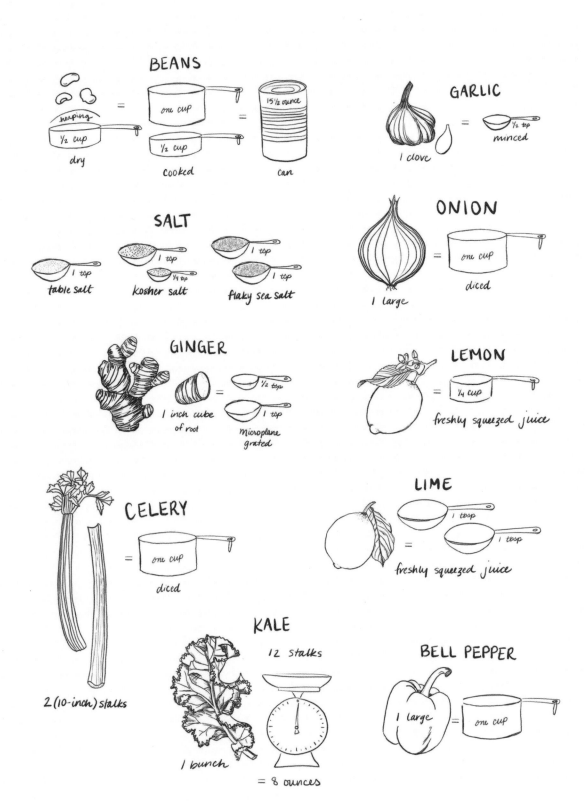

BEANS

heaping ½ cup dry = one cup / ½ cup cooked = 15½ ounce can

GARLIC

1 clove = ½ tsp minced

SALT

1 tsp table salt / 1 tsp + ¼ tsp kosher salt / 1 tsp flaky sea salt

ONION

1 large = one cup diced

GINGER

1 inch cube of root = ½ tbsp / 1 tsp Microplane grated

LEMON

= ¼ cup freshly squeezed juice

CELERY

2 (10-inch) stalks = one cup diced

LIME

= 1 tbsp / 1 tbsp freshly squeezed juice

KALE

1 bunch / 12 stalks = 8 ounces

BELL PEPPER

1 large = one cup

BUTTERNUT SQUASH

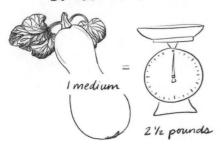

1 medium = 2½ pounds

CHEESE

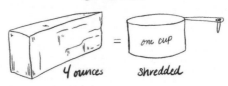

4 ounces = one cup shredded

CORN

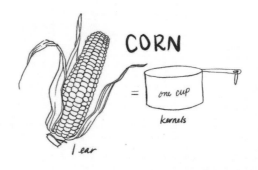

1 ear = one cup kernels

CUCUMBER

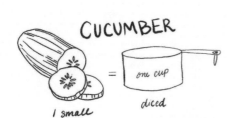

1 small = one cup diced

SALAD GREENS

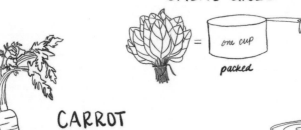

= one cup packed

TOMATO

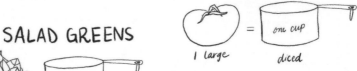

1 large = one cup diced

CARROT

= one cup diced

ZUCCHINI

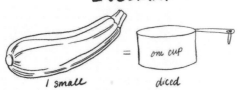

1 small = one cup diced

CANNED TOMATOES

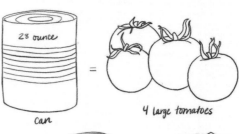

28 ounce can = 4 large tomatoes

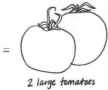

14 ounce can = 2 large tomatoes

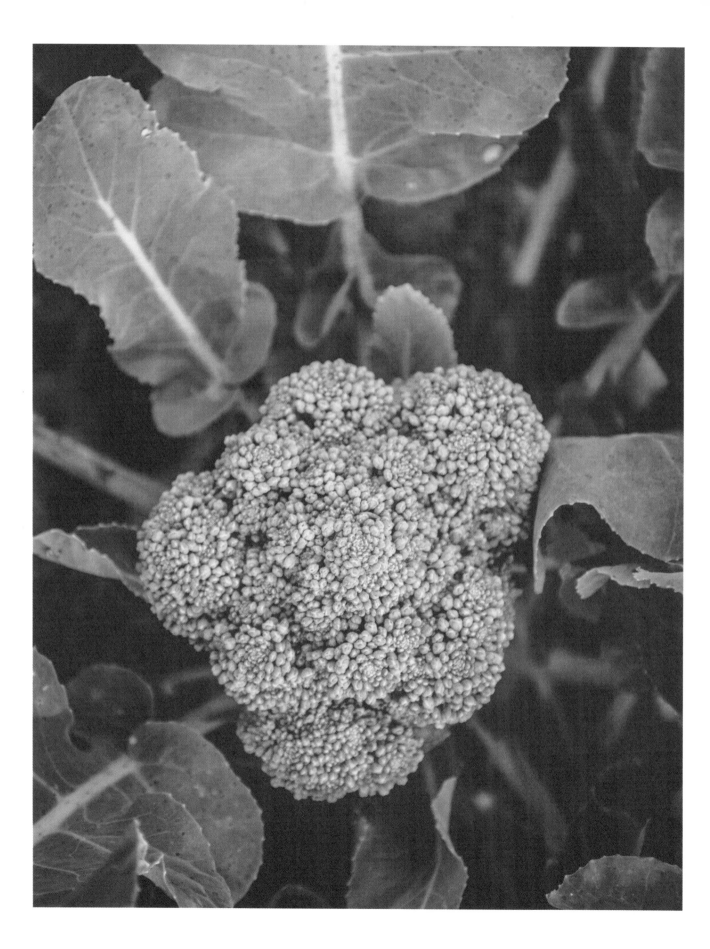

Ingredient Notes

Some of the ingredients used in our recipes may not be familiar to the traditional cook. Here is a guide to what they are, where to find them, and how they are used.

AQUAFABA: The water saved from cooking beans or drained from a can of beans (aqua = water, faba = beans). Aquafaba can add liquid, body, and flavor to a recipe, and it can also be used as a vegan substitute for egg whites in making meringue, with white beans, particularly low sodium chickpeas, yielding best results.

CHIPOTLE PEPPERS IN ADOBO: Chipotles are dried hot chiles (smoked jalapeños) that have been rehydrated and packed in adobo (vinegary tomato sauce). Usually found canned in the international section of grocery stores with the Mexican food items. Making your own is easy if you can get dried chipotle peppers. Try our recipe (p. 279).

COCONUT MILK: The milky liquid from grated coconut pulp. Coconut milk comes in regular or light (less saturated fat; less coconut flavor); you can decide which you prefer to use in these recipes. Coconut milk is a great way to add creaminess without using dairy; however, it does contain saturated fats, which we are advised to consume in moderation for optimal health. For most of us this product is transported great distances (from Indonesia, the Philippines, or India) and comes to us in a can, so use in moderation.

EDAMAME: Green, immature soybeans. Edamame is usually found with the frozen vegetables, either in pods or shelled. It also grows well in gardens. Shelled edamame can be added to a recipe (as you would add frozen corn or peas) for a quick-cooking, mildly nutty-tasting protein. Pods are excellent steamed and served as a snack with a drizzle of olive oil and sprinkle of salt and pepper. Eat just the beans and compost their pods.

FLAXSEED: Waxy seeds, a source of essential omega-3 fats, that must be ground to offer nutritional benefit to the body. You can buy flaxseed already ground or in whole form. We prefer to grind flaxseed ourselves in a spice mill or dedicated coffee grinder. Ground flaxseed loses freshness and nutrients over time, so grind just the amount you need when you need it. Store flaxseed in the refrigerator or freezer for optimal freshness.

FLOUR: Powder that can be made from grains, nuts, or seeds. Flour made from wheat is what people most commonly refer to. We use several varieties of wheat flour in this cookbook:

WHITE FLOURS: Refined to remove bran and germ.

All-Purpose: Milled using a combination of hard and soft wheat for a range of 10–12 percent protein content.

Bread Flour: Made from exclusively hard wheat. Higher in protein, which is desirable in breads for developing gluten and strength.

WHOLE WHEAT FLOURS: Ground from hard wheat using the entire grain, including endosperm, bran, and germ. The bran and germ of whole grains contribute healthy oils, protein, vitamins, minerals, and fiber.

Whole Wheat: Ground from red wheat berries, this is a traditional whole wheat.

White Whole Wheat: Ground from hard white winter wheat, lighter in color and milder in flavor, yet 100 percent whole grain nutrient goodness.

Spelt: An ancient, non-hybrid wheat variety with nutty taste. Dates back to Biblical times (see Exodus 9:32; Isaiah 28:25; Ezekiel 4:9).

Sprouted Wheat: Whole wheat berries misted with water, allowed to sprout, then dried and milled into flour. Sprouting makes nutrients more available.

Whole Grain Flour Blends: Different whole grains that have been milled and blended together. May range from six to twelve grains depending on the manufacturer. Some grains included may be white whole wheat, barley, pumpernickel, sorghum, oat, millet, amaranth, teff, and quinoa flour.

MISO: A fermented soybean paste found in the refrigerated section of grocery stores, typically near the tofu. Used like bouillon to flavor soups, marinades, and dressings. Miso comes in white, yellow, and red varieties. White is the mellowest (fermented for the least amount of time) and red is the strongest and saltiest (fermented the longest).

NUTRITIONAL YEAST: Deactivated yeast that is a nutty, cheesy tasting food product. The same type of yeast used for baking and brewing, except in those applications the yeast is alive; nutritional yeast has been killed with heat. Rich in B vitamins (making it great for vegans looking for a B12 source) and often sprinkled on foods as a cheese substitute. Try it in salad dressings and on popcorn, eggs, mashed potatoes, and pizza. Typically found in the baking aisle, the health food section, or in bulk food sections.

QUINOA: A quick-cooking, high-protein "grain." Quinoa is a seed related to spinach and amaranth and is native to the Andes of South America. Contains all nine essential amino acids, making it a complete protein. Quinoa has a natural coating, called saponin, which has a bitter or soapy taste. Most quinoa in stores has been pre-rinsed to remove this coating, but it doesn't hurt to rinse before use.

SALT: Mineral from evaporated seawater or mined from the earth. There are many types of salt, and none are considered nutritionally superior to another. The size of the grain is what determines how it is used. We keep three types on hand for different purposes: table salt for baking, kosher salt for all-purpose cooking, and flaky sea salt for finishing. Table salt has a fine texture, can pack densely, and thus can be precisely measured, which is desirable when baking. Kosher salt is coarse, making it easy to work with, and dissolves quickly into food. Unlike uniformly shaped table and kosher salt, flaky sea salt is irregular and has a nice finishing touch.

SEITAN: Referred to as "the meat of wheat," seitan is a vegan meat substitute made of gluten, the main protein found in wheat. It is similar to meat in protein content and has a nice chewy texture. Seitan can easily be made from scratch (preferable to avoid extra sodium and other additives) or purchased prepackaged from the grocery store. Found in the refrigerated section next to the tofu or make it yourself using our recipe (p. 195).

TAHINI: A sesame seed paste used in dressings and dips such as hummus. Often found near peanut butter on store shelves. After opening, store in the refrigerator for best shelf life. Making your own is also easy—try our recipe (p. 273).

TEMPEH: A fermented soybean cake that is less processed than tofu. Found refrigerated, usually next to the tofu. Fermentation means that tempeh contains probiotics: good bacteria that provide health benefits. Black spots are a normal sign of fermentation, not spoilage.

TOFU: Soybean curd made in a similar way to cheese. Found refrigerated in grocery stores and comes in silken, firm, and extra firm. Silken tofu is soft and best for blending, such as in a smoothie or dessert. Firm and extra-firm tofu hold shape better for recipes such as a stir-fry.

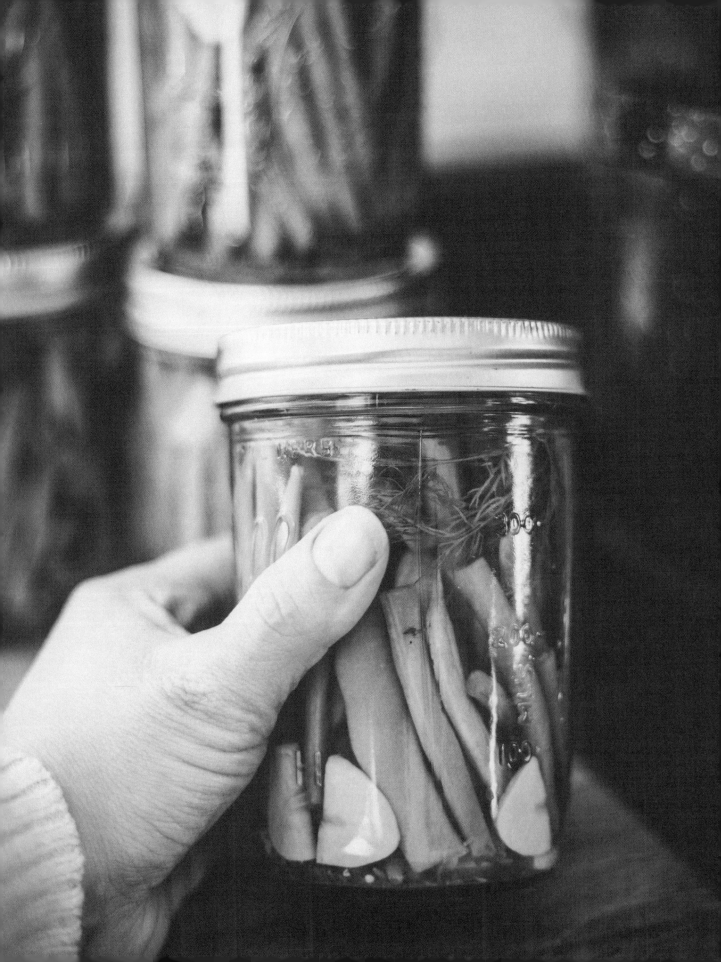

Canning Techniques

Canning is a wonderful way to preserve the harvest. It allows you to store food without electricity, and jars are ready to use right off the shelf. If you are just getting started with canning, you can usually find the equipment needed at a hardware store. Grocery stores often sell jars and lids if you just need to resupply. These instructions are for a method that uses boiling water—also known as water bath canning—rather than for a pressure canning method. Canning times are subject to change according to USDA regulations. For the latest canning times, check your county extension office or the National Center for Home Food Preservation website.

Equipment

- canner with canning rack
- canning jars (pint or quart size depending on your recipe; regular or wide-mouth depending on your preference)
- metal jar rings (also called screw bands, these often come with newly purchased jars; if not, make sure you have a matching ring for each jar you plan to use)
- new canning lids (these often come with newly purchased jars; if reusing jars, purchase new regular or wide-mouth lids to match your jars)

- small, heatproof bowl
- kitchen towel
- clean damp cloth
- jar lifter
- lid lifter magnet (optional)
- ladle
- canning funnel
- bubble tool or chopstick for releasing air

Plan: Determine how much food you plan to can, what size jars you want to use (pints or quarts), and how many jars, rings, and lids you will need. Inspect your jars and remove any with cracks or chips, giving special attention to the rim—both via visual inspection and by running a finger around the jar rim. An imperfection here could lead to a failure to seal.

Prepare jars: Wash and rinse jars and lids. Place the lids in a small, heatproof bowl (you'll be adding hot water to this later). Keep the rings on the counter for now. Place the clean, empty jars on the canning rack inside the canner. Add water, filling and covering the jars with water. Cover the canner, and heat water to just below a boil. Heating the jars now helps prevent the glass from cracking when you add a hot filling or place them back in the boiling water.

You can begin preparing food for canning while the water heats. (Refer now to the specific recipe instructions for what you are canning.)

When food is ready to be packed into jars, use tongs to remove three or four jars from the canner. Carefully tip each jar to dump out the hot water. Pour the water from one of the jars into the heatproof bowl with the lids that you've prepared ahead. The water in the remaining jars can be poured right back into the canner. Set the jars on a kitchen towel.

Proceed with packing the jars according to your recipe instructions. (Refer back to recipe.)

Once jars are packed, use a clean damp cloth to wipe the rim of the jar so there is clean surface for the lid to seal. Use a lid lifter (or tongs or fingers) to remove a lid from the bowl of warm water. Center the lid onto a filled jar. Using only one hand, screw on a rim using just your fingertips to twist. Once the jar starts to twist on the towel, you've got it tight enough. (Some air needs to escape during the processing step, so you don't want lids to be screwed on super tight.) As each jar is filled, use the jar lifter to place it back onto the canner rack in the hot but not boiling water. Repeat with remaining jars.

Can: Once packed, lidded jars are all on the canner rack, proceed with canning in boiling water. Submerge rack of jars fully into the water, making sure jars are covered by 1–2 inches of water. Add more boiling water if needed. Water level should be 2 inches above the jars if processing time is more than 30 minutes (such as for canned tomatoes). Cover the canner and bring to a boil. When the water comes to a full rolling boil, start timing for the minutes required by your specific recipe. A boil must be maintained throughout the entire processing time. (Note: If you live at altitudes above 1,000 feet, you'll need to increase boiling time to account for the lower boiling point: an additional 5 minutes for 1,000–3,000 feet, an additional 10 minutes for 3,001–6,000 feet, and an additional 15 minutes for above 6,000 feet.)

Cool: When boiling-water processing is complete, turn off heat and let jars sit in the hot water for about 5 minutes before removing. This allows the contents of the canner to settle. Then lift the jars out straight with the tongs. Do not tilt! (You may have the urge to dump off the small amount of water pooled on the lid, but the jars must stay upright at this point for best sealing success.) Set them on a dish towel, at least 1 inch apart, for cooling, in a spot where you won't need to move them for a full day and where there isn't a draft. Corners of kitchen counters make nice spots. Allow to cool, undisturbed, for about 24 hours.

Check seal: Now it is time to check your seals. Press down on the center of the lid. If it is down (slightly concave) or stays down, that is a sign of a successful seal. Remove the jar ring. Gently push up on the edge of the lid and see if it stays put. If it does, then your seal is strong and the jar can be stored. Leave the rims off so as not to trap moisture, which can cause rusting. If any jars have not sealed, enjoy eating them immediately or refrigerate to eat within the week.

Store jars: Label and date jars. Store sealed jars in a cool, dark place. Using within the year is recommended, but if you put up a bumper crop, they can last longer than that.

Kitchen Techniques

These techniques are used frequently in our recipes, so we thought it a good idea to share some tips that will help you be efficient, safe, and successful in the kitchen.

BLENDING HOT SOUP: Use an immersion blender to avoid having to pour a hot liquid. To safely puree a hot soup using a traditional blender or food processor, blend in batches, only filling halfway and removing the center insert of the lid for venting. Hold a kitchen towel over the opening to prevent splattering.

BLOOMING SPICES: Cooking spices briefly in oil releases fat-soluble flavor compounds. It makes them, by some estimates, ten times more flavorful, and it allows them to "bloom"—to have flavors be distributed more evenly throughout a dish.

CARING FOR CAST IRON: Cast iron makes for great cookware. Yes, it is heavy, but it will last a lifetime. Cast iron takes a bit longer to heat up, but once it does, it has great heat retention and even heat. Most cast iron comes pre-seasoned, which makes it virtually nonstick naturally. Maintaining cast iron need not be intimidating. After use, wash with hot water and mild soap only if needed. Stuck-on food can be removed by scrubbing with a mix of kosher salt and water. Dry the cast iron immediately after washing to prevent rust spots. Rub a light coating of oil on the surface and heat on a burner over medium heat for a minute or two. Now it is ready for its next cooking job.

If you need to rehab an abused pan, here is how to strip and restore: Remove any light rust with fine steel wool (severe rust might need machine grinding to remove). Wash with water and mild soap, using a bristle brush. Dry. Lightly oil everywhere, including handle and bottom of pan. Place upside down in a 350°F oven for 1 hour. Remove. Let cool. Wipe the pan down, and ideally, repeat with another light coating of oil, heating, cooling. You are now ready to cook with reclaimed cast iron. When storing, it is best to not stack any pot or pan, especially cast iron.

COMPOSTING: Keep food scraps out of the landfill by composting. (Note: This is guidance about making regular composting deposits and not inclusive of instructions for initial setup of a pile/bin or capping it when it is full.) Have a small pail in a convenient spot in your kitchen, such as under the sink or on the countertop, where you can deposit scraps. What can go into your pail? Think of it as vegetarian: no meat, bones, or dairy. Also avoid grease. Empty your pail regularly either at a facility that accepts food scraps or in a backyard compost pile or bin. If you can compost at home, you need more than just food scraps to make good soil. Compost without browns is just rotting food. Compost needs air, and browns help provide that. A recipe of 3 parts brown (carbon material) to 1 part green/food scraps (nitrogen material) is ideal. Each time you make a deposit of green food scraps, pull back the old brown material to the edges, making a new center nest. Add the food scraps to the middle and cover with new brown material using the 3:1 ratio. A good rule of thumb is to have brown all around. This optimizes the carbon-to-nitrogen ratio and prevents odor (odor is what attracts animals). Compost that is too wet has a strong odor and needs more browns mixed in. Keep a supply of mixed dry browns from a variety of materials near your compost pile/bin in a separate bin or trash can so that it is easy to access each time you empty your kitchen scraps. Too much brown material and your pile will be slow to break down.

WHAT TO COMPOST

BROWNS (CARBON): DEAD, VERY DRY MATERIALS PROVIDE AIR CARBOHYDRATES/ENERGY FOR SOIL MICROBES	GREENS (NITROGEN): LIVING, WET MATERIALS PROVIDE WATER PROTEIN FOR SOIL MICROBES
DRY LEAVES, PINE NEEDLES	FRUIT AND VEGETABLE SCRAPS*
HOUSEHOLD PAPER PRODUCTS: CARDBOARD ROLLS, BOX BOARD, EGG CARTONS, NEWSPAPER, PAPER BAGS, PAPER TOWELS, TISSUE PAPER, NON-GLOSSY PAPER, TOOTHPICKS, CORKS, MATCHES	COFFEE GROUNDS AND TEA LEAVES
	GRAINS AND BEANS
	VEGETARIAN LEFTOVERS
	FLOWER CUTTINGS, GARDEN PLANTS
STRAW	WEEDS THAT HAVEN'T GONE TO SEED
SAWDUST, SMALL WOOD CHIPS	HAY
COFFEE FILTERS AND TEA BAGS (REMOVE STAPLES)	DRY GRASS CLIPPINGS (MIXED WITH OTHER INGREDIENTS BEFORE ADDING TO PREVENT CLUMPING)
NATURAL FIBERS: BAMBOO, COTTON, LEATHER, LINEN, SILK, WOOL	MANURE FROM HERBIVORES
DRYER LINT (NATURAL FIBERS ONLY)	CRUSHED EGGSHELLS (A MINERAL, SO TECHNICALLY NEITHER GREEN OR BROWN)

*Remember to remove all stickers from produce peels before composting.

Note: Smaller pieces will compost quicker: Shred or break up brown materials. Cut up green materials. "Compostable" plates, cups, utensils, and bags may be very slow to break down in backyard bins/piles. Opt for reusable or paper products.

COOKING WHOLE GRAINS: There are several methods for cooking grains. First, sort them using the same technique described on page 313 for dry beans and lentils.

STOVETOP METHOD: Bring liquid and grain to a boil. Add a pinch or two of salt if desired. Reduce heat to low. Cover tightly and simmer until done cooking. Drain off excess water. Fluff grains with a fork. Recover and allow to sit for about 5 minutes before serving.

"Pasta" method: This only works for larger grains (not amaranth, millet, quinoa, or teff). Double the water called for in the stovetop method but cook the same length of time, draining off excess water when done. This eliminates the risk of burning in your pot as the water simmers out.

PRESSURE-COOKING: Reduces cooking time significantly. Cook on high pressure followed by a 10-minute natural release. This method is reserved for larger grains with longer cook times (once again, not amaranth, millet, quinoa, or teff).

MEASURES AND COOK TIMES FOR WHOLE GRAINS

WHOLE GRAIN (1 CUP)	WATER (CUPS)	STOVETOP COOKING TIME (MINUTES)	PRESSURE-COOKING TIME (MINUTES)
AMARANTH	3	20	N/A
BARLEY*	3	60	35
BROWN RICE	2 (1¼ for pressure-cooking)	40	20
FARRO*	2	60	30
KAMUT (KHORASAN WHEAT)	3	60	30
MILLET, HULLED	3	20	N/A
OAT GROATS	3	60	30
QUINOA	2	15	N/A
RYE BERRIES	3½	60	30
SPELT BERRIES	3	60	30
TEFF	4	15	N/A
WHEAT BERRIES	3	60	30

*Barley and farro cook times given here are for whole, hulled forms. Frequently what is sold in the store is either a pearled or semi-pearled form. Hulled grains have only the outermost hull removed, retaining nutrients and fiber. Pearled or semi-pearled grains are polished to remove the bran layer. They are softer and have fewer nutrients but cook in about half the time.

CUTTING VEGETABLES: There is a lot of vegetable cutting in a vegetarian cookbook! There are many different ways to cut your vegetables, and each term has a specific definition. When you are familiar with the various cuts called for, recipes will turn out better.

CHIFFONADE: rolled, thinly sliced

CHOP: casual, not a precise or uniform cut

DICE: large ¾ inch (roasting); medium ½ inch (soups, stews); small ¼ inch (quick-cooking sauté or stir-fry). *Note:* In this cookbook, instructions to dice assume a medium dice. When we want a small dice size, we specify to finely dice. For large dice, we specify a ¾-inch cut.

JULIENNE: thin strips, sometimes referred to as matchstick cuts, about ⅛ x ⅛ x 1 or 2 inches long

MINCE: small, random

DRAINING AND RINSING CANNED BEANS: Canned foods can have high salt content. Emptying a can of beans into a colander and rinsing under water has been shown to reduce sodium by 40 percent. This technique also removes some indigestible compounds, thereby decreasing flatulence.

GRINDING NUTS, SEEDS, AND SPICES: When a food is ground (such as for flour, nut or seed butters, flaxseed, or any spices), it becomes exposed to air and will start to lose flavor and nutrient potency. It is best to use up ground spices within a year for best flavor. Replace anything not used up after 3 years. Some stores offer bulk spices; you can purchase just what you need of a spice that you might not use often. Ideally, grind your own as needed. Have a dedicated coffee or spice grinder just for grinding up fresh, small batches of nuts, seeds, whole grains, and spices. To care for your grinder: Clean the hopper after each use with a dry bristle brush (washing with water is not recommended, as it can seep into the motor and cause it to short out). Occasionally clean out the oily residue by putting ¼ cup dry whole grain (such as rice, barley, or wheat berries) into the hopper, grinding it up into a flour, then brushing it out and wiping clean. Compost the flour when cleaning is complete.

MEASURING FLOUR: Be precise when measuring your flour for baking to achieve best results.

TO MEASURE BY VOLUME: Fluff up flour with a spoon, then gently sift spoonfuls into your measuring cup, using a light touch. Once the cup is mounded full, use a flat edge to scrape across the top of the cup, leveling it.

TO MEASURE BY WEIGHT: You will need to use a kitchen scale. This is the most precise and preferred method for measuring flour. This weight conversion chart, which we created for this cookbook, is based on 1 cup of King Arthur brand flour (a local-to-us, employee-owned B Corp) unless noted otherwise.

FLOUR MEASURES BY WEIGHT

FLOUR (1 CUP)	GRAM WEIGHT
ALL-PURPOSE	123
BREAD	123
SPELT (BOB'S RED MILL)	117
SPROUTED WHEAT	111
WHITE WHOLE WHEAT	127
WHOLE WHEAT	127
WHOLE GRAIN FLOUR BLEND (9-GRAIN)	115

MISE EN PLACE: A technique of having everything in place when you cook, making for a more efficient and enjoyable experience in the kitchen. French for "putting in place," mise en place encompasses having an organized kitchen space and arranging the tools and ingredients that your recipe calls for before starting. Keeping a clean workspace is very important. Clean as you go, keeping workspaces clear and tools ready for reuse. Mise en place is also a mindset: thinking through the use of your time, being organized with what you plan to prepare. Time, space, and resources are precious, so have a plan to be efficient and use them well.

PREHEATING THE OVEN: Most recipes are written with directions to preheat the oven. But now that we are more attentive to energy use and conservation practices, we can question the need to preheat every time a recipe requires the oven. Baking anything that requires a lift (via yeast, baking soda, baking powder) does best in a preheated oven. Almost everything else—vegetables, casseroles, mixed dishes—doesn't. Simply start them in a cold oven and lengthen your baking time by about 5 minutes. This practice will add up to be an energy saver, especially in those times when the oven preheats well ahead of when you are ready to use it. Then again, if your oven has been on for other things and you want to make something of ours that calls for a cold oven, there's no need to wait for it to cool. In that case, it is most efficient to use the already preheated oven and reduce the cook time by 5 minutes. There is also no need to stir partway through cooking unless you prefer even browning, which will occur more on the bottom side. The less frequently you open the oven, the less heat escapes.

PRESSING TOFU: Removes excess water, which then allows the tofu to absorb more flavors from other ingredients in the recipe. Press tofu by wrapping it up in a clean kitchen towel, then place a weight, such as a heavy pot or several books on a plate, on top. Leave tofu under the weight for at least 20 minutes.

ROASTING VEGETABLES: The recipes in this book frequently include roasting vegetables. Roasting at a high temperature, with a touch of oil and seasonings, transforms what could otherwise be boiled and bland into caramelized, irresistible treats popular with kids and grown-up veggie skeptics alike. The flavor that develops by using this method—cooking veggies at a high heat—seems worth it. Since it is an energy-intensive method, try to plan ahead and be ready to cook multiple things that require the oven. You could fill all the oven racks with vegetables, for example, and enjoy leftovers throughout the week. Here are a few tips:

- Use a dark pan, as this will absorb and reflect more heat, which promotes browning. If you are roasting with a sweetener (honey or maple syrup), you can use parchment paper for ease of cleanup and still get some browning. Do not use a silicone baking mat, as this would inhibit browning.

- Cut vegetables so they are uniform in size; this will ensure they cook evenly. About 1 inch is a nice size for roasting.

- Choose a high-heat oil (an oil with a high smoke point). Regular olive oil is our go-to oil for roasting.

- Spread vegetables in a single layer. This helps ensure even cooking and good caramelization.

- Stirring is optional. The cut side facing down on the baking sheet is what will caramelize/brown most. If you want even browning, stir once halfway through. If you prefer one side be very caramelized, don't stir.

TOASTING NUTS AND SEEDS: This is an optional but highly recommended step in our recipes, as it draws out the natural oils, adding to the flavor. It doesn't take long, and the difference in taste is noticeable. There are several ways to toast: on the stovetop, when you need just a handful toasted quickly; in the oven, when you have a lot of nuts to toast and want even browning, or in the microwave. No additional oil is needed, as the natural oils are enough to prevent sticking.

STOVETOP: Place nuts or seeds in a dry skillet over medium-low heat, stirring often until golden brown and fragrant, no more than 5 minutes. Remove from skillet immediately and let cool.

OVEN: Spread nuts or seeds on a baking sheet in a single layer. Place in a cold oven and turn to 350°F. Start timing and bake for 10–15 minutes, or until toasted golden brown. Remove from baking sheet immediately and let cool.

MICROWAVE: Place nuts or seeds on a microwaveable plate. Cook on high for 3 minutes, pausing to stir halfway through. Remove from plate immediately and let cool.

MEASURING: A heaping ½ cup dry beans will yield 1½ cups cooked beans, equivalent to 1 (15½-ounce) can. A heaping 1 cup dry beans will yield 3 cups cooked beans, equivalent to 2 (15½-ounce) cans. One pound dry beans is equal to 2½ cups dry beans.

SORTING AND RINSING: Spread onto a rimmed baking sheet in a single layer and shake gently side to side. Remove any broken pieces and foreign items, such as small pebbles, pieces of pod, or hulls. Rinse in a fine-mesh sieve or colander. This technique also applies to sorting lentils and whole grains.

SOAKING: Soaking dry beans rehydrates them and removes some indigestible compounds that contribute to flatulence. There are three methods:

traditional (overnight) soak: This method is preferred if you will be cooking the beans in a pressure cooker. In a large bowl, cover the beans in water and let them soak overnight, or at least 8 hours. If you live in a warm climate, soak beans in the refrigerator to prevent fermentation. There should be about 1 inch of water above the top of the beans. Drain, rinse, and proceed with cooking.

hot soak: This method is preferred over the quick soak if time allows. Place beans in a pot with water (5 cups water for every 1 cup beans). Bring to a boil and cook for 2–3 minutes. Turn off heat, cover, and let sit for 4–24 hours. Drain, rinse, and proceed with cooking.

quick soak: This is the same as the hot soak method but with less water and less time. Place beans in a saucepot with water (3 cups water for every 1 cup beans). Bring to a boil and cook for 2–3 minutes. Turn off heat, cover, and let sit for 1 hour. Drain, rinse, and proceed with cooking.

COOKING:

traditional boil: Cook beans in a large, covered pot. Use fresh, cold water to a depth of 1 inch above the beans. Bring to a boil. Reduce heat and simmer gently until beans are tender. Stir occasionally and add warm water if needed to keep the beans covered throughout the cooking time. Cook time will vary by the bean.

pressure-cook: Will reduce cooking time significantly. Place soaked beans in the pressure cooker. Cover with enough water so that it is 1 inch above the beans. Cook on high pressure. Time will vary by the bean. Use a natural release method (let the pressure cooker sit for about 10 minutes after it finishes cooking before opening).

Cooking times for soaked beans vary.

COOKING TIMES FOR SOAKED DRY BEANS

BEAN	BOILING (HOURS)	PRESSURE-COOKING (MINUTES)
BLACK BEAN	1–1½	5–8
BLACK-EYED PEA	1	4
CANNELLINI	1–1½	5–8
CHICKPEA	1½–2	11–14
GREAT NORTHERN	1	5–8
NAVY	1½	5–8
PINTO	1½	5–8
RED KIDNEY	1½	5–8
SOLDIER	1½	5–8

- Salt (1 teaspoon per pound of beans) added to cooking water can add flavor and prevent beans from getting mushy.

- Oil (1 tablespoon per pound of beans) added to cooking water can add creaminess and decrease foaming during cooking.

- Old beans, peas, and lentils will take longer to cook, so if your legumes aren't softened by the suggested cook time, it may be that they've exceeded their shelf life.

STORING: Storing beans in their cooking liquid (aquafaba) will keep them tender and flavorful. Beans freeze well for later use, so cook up plenty when you have the time. Freeze them in quantities called for in recipes. For example, 1½ cups cooked beans covered by cooking liquid will be equal to 1 (15½-ounce) can.

Notes

1 Walter Willett et al., "Food in the Anthropocene: The EAT-Lancet Commission on Healthy Diets from Sustainable Food Systems," The Lancet 393, no. 10170 (February 2, 2019): 447–92, www.thelancet.com/journals/lancet/article/PIIS0140-6736(18)31788-4/fulltext.

2 "Leading Causes of Death," National Center for Health Statistics, Centers for Disease Control and Prevention, last modified March 12, 2017, www.cdc.gov/nchs/fastats/leading-causes-of-death.htm.

3 "Preventing Chronic Diseases: A Vital Investment," Chronic Diseases and Health Promotion, World Health Organization, accessed May 28, 2019, www.who.int/chp/chronic_disease_report/part1/en/index11.html.

4 "Choose My Plate," United States Department of Agriculture, accessed May 20, 2019, https://www.choosemyplate.gov/.

5 "2015–2020 Dietary Guidelines for Americans, 8th Edition," U.S. Department of Health and Human Services and U.S. Department of Agriculture, December 2015, www.health.gov/dietaryguidelines/2015/guidelines/.

6 Preamble to the Constitution of the World Health Organization, 1948, available at https://www.who.int/governance/eb/who_constitution_en.pdf.

7 "2018 Was 4th Hottest Year on Record for the Globe," National Oceanic and Atmospheric Association, last modified February 26, 2019, www.noaa.gov/news/2018-was-4th-hottest-year-on-record-for-globe; "GISS Surface Temperature Analysis (v3)," National Aeronautics and Space Administration, last modified May 15, 2019, https://data.giss.nasa.gov/gistemp/graphs/.

8 Kari Hamerschlag, "Meat Eaters' Guide to Climate Change," (Environmental Working Group, July 2011), 6, https://static.ewg.org/reports/2011/meateaters/pdf/report_ewg_meat_eaters_guide_to_health_and_climate_2011.pdf.

9 "Total Red Meat and Poultry, Livestock and Meat Domestic Data, All Supply and Disappearance," United States Department of Agriculture (USDA), Economic Research Service (ERS), last modified April 26, 2019, www.ers.usda.gov/data-products/livestock-meat-domestic-data/livestock-meat-domestic-data/#All_supply_and_disappearance.

10 "Meat Consumption," Organization for Economic Co-operation and Development, 2018, https://data.oecd.org/agroutput/meat-consumption.htm.

11 Intergovernmental Panel on Climate Change, AR5 Climate Change 2014: Mitigation of Climate Change (Cambridge University Press, 2014), 24, www.ipcc.ch/report/ar5/wg3/.

12 Dana Gunders, "Wasted: How America Is Losing Up to 40 Percent of Its Food from Farm to Fork to Landfill," (New York: Natural Resources Defense Council, 2012), www.nrdc.org/sites/default/files/wasted-food-IP.pdf.

13 United States Environmental Protection Agency, "Advancing Sustainable Materials Management: 2015 Fact Sheet," (Washington, DC: EPA, 2018), https://www.epa.gov/sites/production/files/2018-07/documents/2015_smm_msw_factsheet_07242018_fnl_508_002.pdf.

14 Walter Willett et al., "Food in the Anthropocene: The EAT-Lancet Commission on Healthy Diets from Sustainable Food Systems," The Lancet 393, no. 10170 (February 2, 2019): 447–92, www.thelancet.com/journals/lancet/article/PIIS0140-6736(18)31788-4/fulltext.

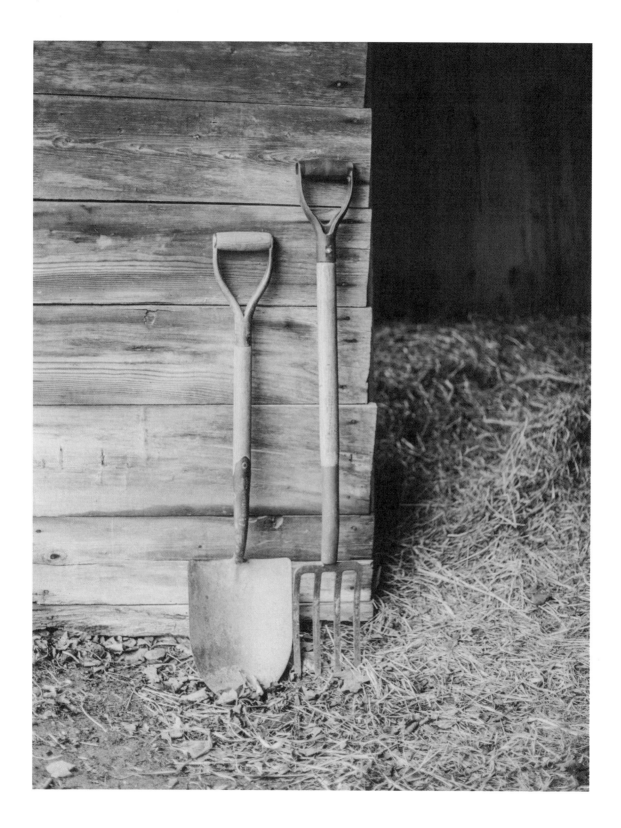

Acknowledgments

We want to offer our sincere gratitude for everyone who has been involved in this project.

First, we want to thank our immediate families—Steve, Jacob, and Silas McCloskey, and Nick, Norah, Helen, and Esther Wolfe—for their time as we put this idea in writing for the publisher and then all the hours of recipe planning, testing, writing, photography, and design (though we don't think they minded the recipe-testing phase too much).

We had additional recipe testers scattered all over the United States. Thank you to Nancy Wolfe, Elizabeth Fox, Holly Pascoe, Katie Wheel, Heather Kulp, Mary Guntz, Laura Beidler, Rachel and Adam Barehl, Marcos Stoltzfus, Margaret Apura, Monica Bergquist, Janice Zook, Dave and Carmeleta Beidler, Valerie Brewer, Jane Glick, Jennifer Schrock, Rachel Shields, Brenda Metzler, Ruth Ellen Dandurand, Amber Bergey, and Jenn Driscoll. Their thoughtful feedback helped us refine the recipe collection you now hold in your hands.

We are most appreciative of our supportive families and friends who believed in us and our cause, including Laura and Tom Grothe; Sarah, Stephen, Isaac, and Rae Donovan; Gerry and Karen Hawkes; Norman and Nancy Wolfe; and our entire church congregation at Taftsville Chapel Mennonite Fellowship in Vermont. We are grateful for their frequent recipe testing at family gatherings, church potlucks, and coffee times, and for being sounding boards as we formulated our thoughts around food and faith, preparing to write the front matter for this book.

A special thanks to a group self-labeled as a "discernment circle," of which Jaynie was a member along with Rachel Ebersole, Sarah Allen, and Courtney Hollingsworth. Additional thanks to Amanda Barnhart, who helped via phone and email to process the book idea during this time as well.

Thanks to Steve Kriss, who sat with the McCloskey family over lunch, heard this book's elevator pitch, and enthusiastically connected us with Herald Press. We are grateful to our publishing team at Herald Press, particularly Valerie Weaver-Zercher, who gave us the opportunity to make this book possible.

Thanks to the very talented Rachel Joy Barehl for the lifestyle photography and some food photography scattered throughout these pages. And thank you to Ruth Ann Glick and Carie Good for lending photography props for our initial photography proposal to Herald Press. Our gratitude to the Fox family at High Low Farm for outfitting and educating us about beekeeping while we took photos. Thanks to Allison Good for writing out the music to our family prayer songs and to master composter Cat Buxton for lending her expertise.

Additionally, Heather wishes to extend appreciation to her employer, Dartmouth-Hitchcock, and specifically to her colleagues on the employee wellness team, who have supported her interest in culinary medicine and provided a platform for developing her skills as a recipe writer.

Last, but not least, we'd like to thank local businesses: Farmhouse Pottery and Simon Pierce, for the use of their artisan pottery and glassware in our photography; the Upper Valley Food Co-op, for letting us take photos of where we shop locally for whole, healthy, and fair foods; the Apple Hill Inn, for the use of their beautiful barn that neighbors our chapel and was where all our local testers convened for a celebration of our project in thanks for their support; and the Bridgewater Thrift Shop, for donating thirty-two gorgeous place settings of eclectic dinnerware for the barn party.

Index

The Authors

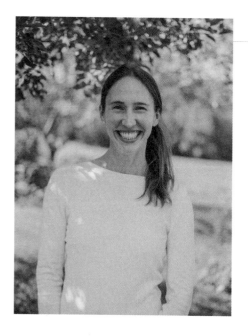

Heather Wolfe is a registered dietitian nutritionist and certified health coach at Dartmouth-Hitchcock. Wolfe earned a bachelor of science degree in dietetics, nutrition, and food sciences from the University of Vermont and a master of public health degree from the Geisel School of Medicine at Dartmouth. She has been providing nutrition counseling and health coaching for over 15 years, mostly in employee wellness, helping people discover the knowledge, skills, habits, and motivation needed to eat well and be well. Wolfe is a food enthusiast and homesteader who enjoys permaculture gardening, scratch cooking, and raising backyard chickens in Vermont alongside her husband and three daughters.

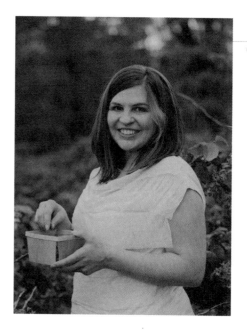

Jaynie McCloskey is a Graphic Designer with a degree in fine arts from The Ohio State University. She attributes her culinary guidance to a wide variety of cookbook authors and food bloggers she's followed over the past 12 years. McCloskey has found cooking plant-based meals to be healing, for both body and soul. She also enjoys exploring Vermont hiking trails and local farm-to-table cafés with her family and friends.